Here are just some of the moving and heartfelt testimonials for *Love Yourself Thin*.

"You write as though you are talking to me and about me like no one else could ever do before."

—J. G., Nevada

"Thank you for writing *Love Yourself Thin*. I am thankful I have such knowledge."

—E. B., Colorado

"This book makes every diet book I've read before seem like a Band-Aid."

—L. M., New York

"Thank you for this marvelous book. For the first time in my 38 years, I am free. I love you for awakening in me what seemed so impossible before."

—S. S., California

"*Love Yourself Thin* has made such a wonderful difference in my life. I have a better relationship with myself and no longer have the tremendous sense of struggle over weight issues."

—C. E., Connecticut

"Victoria shares herself and her knowledge in a way that makes it easy to take her advice."

—L. L., California

"I have had difficulty for 30 years struggling with being overweight. Not only did *Love Yourself Thin* open up the idea that I might look at loving myself sufficiently, but the recipes are incredible."

—E. F., Texas

"Thank you very much for giving me a lot of practical advice and tips, for feeding my spirit with the love that obviously went into the writing, for giving me so many rich and beautiful examples of ageless wisdom, and for all the great recipes!"

—D. J., Kansas

"Your book has helped me immensely in ways I can't explain. I've read it and reread it, and it always touches me. I feel I'm definitely dealing with my overeating problem; I know I've come a long way."

—A. G., Ontario, Canada

LOVE
YOURSELF
THIN

LOVE YOURSELF THIN

THE REVOLUTIONARY SPIRITUAL APPROACH TO WEIGHT LOSS

Victoria Moran

Recipes by Sonnet Pierce

DAYBREAK™ BOOKS
AN IMPRINT OF RODALE BOOKS
NEW YORK, NEW YORK

NOTICE

This book is intended as a reference volume only, not as a medical manual. The information given here is designed to help you make informed decisions about your health. It is not intended as a substitute for any treatment that may have been prescribed by your doctor. If you suspect that you have a medical problem, we urge you to seek competent medical help.

TO RACHAEL

Thanks for your patience for sharing more than two years
of your childhood with this project.
For any good this book does, at least half the credit is yours.

CONTENTS

ACKNOWLEDGMENTS

I wish to thank my agent Patti Breitman for bringing this work to the attention of the publisher; my editor Karen Kelly for believing in the book and for all her hard work; Sonnet Pierce for her wonderful recipes (and for all the nights I didn't have to cook because she brought dishes over for us to sample); George Eisman, R.D., Suzanne Havala, R.D., and Michael Klaper, M.D., for their nutritional expertise; the Vegetarian Resource Group for their help on the list of vegetarian celebrities. I would also like to thank all those who filled out questionnaires concerning their recovery from food addictions as well as the hundreds of recovering people who have guided and inspired me over the years; Alcoholics Anonymous and Overeaters Anonymous for the wisdom of the Twelve Steps; everyone who read this book in its first incarnation as *The Love-Powered Diet* and wrote to me to tell me how it made a difference for them; Marilyn Diamond for her encouragement to write what was in my heart; and to my friends Helene Martin Lynn, Diann Roche, Suzanne Tague, and Carol Shiflett, in particular, who always told me this book would have another life.

AUTHOR'S NOTE

The premise of *Love Yourself Thin* is simple. It is one idea that has two parts.

1. Inner awareness of unconditional Love can make profound changes in a person's life.
2. Inner change includes the ability to make positive, loving food choices.

This book is especially addressed to food addicts—that is, any person of any body size who is engaged in a long-standing battle with a knife and fork. Its principles can, however, help anyone eat more healthfully and live more happily.

The format of the Twelve Steps, originally developed by Alcoholics Anonymous, is used in this book. These steps are not the only way to bring about a spiritual awakening powerful enough to change one's life and behavior, but they have had unparalleled success in helping people with a wide range of dependencies, including alcohol, drugs, unhealthy relationships, and compulsive eating. There is no official or unofficial connection between this book and any Twelve Step organization.

The loving food choices referred to involve selecting natural foods that promote physical health and discourage overeating. Choosing these foods expresses Love not only to oneself but also to the world in general, including non-human animals and the environment. Connecting this way of eating to a Twelve Step lifestyle is my idea. Neither Overeaters Anonymous nor any other Twelve Step group that I know of endorses any particular dietary choice.

The spiritual and physical aspects of loving yourself thin, however, are two sides of a single whole. There are many people who have overcome eating disorders by approaching food differently than I suggest. Nevertheless, linking the two creates a winning combination. In fact, one can lead to the other. A person who deepens his or her spiritual life often evolves toward a gentler, more natural diet. Conversely, people who improve their diets, particularly those who become vegetarians, are often led to explore their spiritual natures.

Recognizing that spirituality is an emotionally charged subject for many people, I have done my best to keep my vocabulary and references nonthreatening both to people who are religious and to those who are not. If there are any references in this book that make you uncomfortable, please substitute a word, phrase, or concept that is comfortable for you, such as "Love" for "God." You do not have to change your beliefs about religion or an afterlife to draw upon the Love already within you and make this life one of freedom and joy.

To be informed when Victoria Moran will be in your area, or to host a *Love Yourself Thin* workshop, write to the author at P. O. Box 3344, Kansas City, KS 66103.

Introduction

T HIS IS YOUR FAIRY GODMOTHER SPEAKING. You can have a body that you think is gorgeous—not just for the ball, but forever. You can go to sleep at night without hating yourself for what you ate during the day, and you'll never again need to count calories or carbohydrates, grams of fat, or ounces of food. You only need to count yourself lucky for having discovered how to love yourself thin.

Okay, so I'm not your fairy godmother. I'm another person just like you with a food problem that took me around the block so many times I could have passed as a meter reader. I cannot zap you with a magic wand. You'll just think that I did once you discover within yourself a source of power to change your eating and your life—one that's more effective than a regiment of fairy godmothers marching in formation. This is the power of Love. Don't be put off by an overused word. It is an extremely underused resource.

You know how being in Love transforms the way in which people look and feel and how loving someone or something—even a goldfish or a parakeet—can give a person a sense of worth and purpose. There's more than one story about a small woman lifting an automobile off her child trapped beneath it. There is also abundant evidence of the crucial role that Love plays in healing. Physicians such as Bernie Siegel, Larry Dossey, and C. Norman Shealy have documented in numerous books how loving oneself and others can mean the difference between getting well and giving up. When patients open themselves to Love as an active energy in its own right, they can experience changes in their own bodies and emotions that appear miraculous. You may think of this as divine Love, or as the synchronizing force that keeps electrons whirling about the nucleus of every atom.

1

No matter how you perceive it, this Love can revolutionize your relationship with food. This is because the Love already inside you is not only strengthening and healing, it is filling. If you have a history of overeating and being overweight—or its flip side of chronic dieting, bulimia, or compulsive exercising—you may have already realized that you're not eating to fill your stomach. You're eating to fill a gash in your soul as devastating to your well-being as the one in the ozone could be to this planet. It's what French philosopher Blaise Pascal called the God-shaped hole in every man that only God can fill.

There is not enough food on Earth to fill that inner void, and there are not enough friends, lovers, or children; houses, cars, or stock certificates; clothes, compliments, or accomplishments to fill it either. Nevertheless, when you connect with Love, a comfortable sense of "enoughness" begins to emerge. Popular dictionaries don't recognize enoughness as a word, but without it, you and food will always be at war. You win this battle when you refuse to fight. Attach your willpower to the nearest white flag and let Love take over. That's when you will understand that *you* are enough. You are attractive enough. You are lovable enough. And for this day, the most important one right now, you are thin enough. When I use the word *thin*, I don't mean model thin or athlete thin or adolescent thin. I mean feeling comfortable with your body and proud to walk around in it. Thin, as used in this book, means having a body that serves you well so you can live freely without wishing you weighed less.

Do you know what will happen when you comprehend—not just with your head but with your heart and your spirit—that you are indeed thin enough for the day at hand, that you are truly attractive and lovable? You will treat yourself as someone who is all those things. For starters, you'll eat like a thin, attractive, lovable person does. When I was fighting food with the vigor of a fresh Marine recruit, a wise old fellow told me that I was putting the cart before the horse in trying to eat less than I wanted and exercise more. He said that it works the other way around, that people who are healthy automatically do healthy things.

Goodness knows, I was an authority on healthy things. I had been writing articles about health, fitness, and beauty since I was 19. I read, researched, and wrote, keeping abreast of the latest trends in diet, nutrition, exercise, and behavior modification. I interviewed experts and passed their findings along. I had accumulated so much information that my head ached, but I was trapped in a binge/diet cycle so insidious that most of the time, my heart ached, too. It was embarrassing enough to go from fat to thin and back again like a human accordion. In addition to seeing myself as a diet failure, I saw myself as a phony. The words I wrote were true based on the knowledge available at the time, but I wasn't able to put them into practice. Like a marriage counselor going through his fifth divorce, my work and my life were sorely fragmented.

Fragmentation—fragmented lives in a fragmented society—is a component most of the time when eating is out of balance. Loving yourself thin meets fragmentation with integration because pure, essential Love is an integrating force. It doesn't foster bits and pieces. Love will not only make a difference in what you eat or the amount of exercise you get but it will also enhance the way you feel about your body. The integrating power of Love can bring all your parts into a functioning whole. When it infuses the way you eat and the way you live, your body will definitely show results, but so will every other aspect of your life. Nothing less than that can bring about changes that last.

When Love fills your emptiness and integrates your fragmented factions, you'll no longer need a closet filled with clothes that range in sizes from those found at the petite boutique to those found at the stout shop. You won't need to be a person who starts every Monday with a dismal diet that is tossed aside by Tuesday afternoon. You can stop spending your money on every pill, potion, and promise that comes around. The kind of Love I'm talking about keeps its promises a day at a time, just as surely as the sun brings light every morning. Without that, weight loss is destined to be temporary. You know that's as true as an oath in court because you've lost weight before. You'd be better off keeping the body you have right now and learning to cherish it than to have one more raving success with a diet, then blow the lid off it and despise yourself. Those episodes erode the spirit. You deserve the chance to leave them behind for good.

The only way I know to bring destructive eating to a screeching halt and to keep it there on a daily basis is to let Love handle it. I not only tried the other ways but I also wrote articles about them. There were plenty of good ideas in these approaches. Many were sane and logical, devised by intelligent and compassionate people, but the power to make them work for me wasn't there. They presented valid facts about nutrition or exercise or "thinking thin," but these facts were as useless to me as one perfectly decent battery in a flashlight that needs two.

Loving yourself thin is different because it works on both perspective and practice. On an inner level, it means trading willpower for Love's power. In practical application, it means living and eating in Love-inspired fashion. The foods you'll prefer will be those that express Love—to your physical self, to all living-kind, and to the planet that provides our food in the first place. You won't be dieting. It has been recognized at long last that regimentation cannot realistically be imposed on natural processes, and that responding to hunger is as natural as blinking or breathing. Instead of dieting, you will be choosing to care for yourself and those around you as you make your selections at the supermarket and from the restaurant menu.

Because you're worth the best, your way of eating will reflect the low-fat, high-fiber, and high-carbohydrate recommendations of the surgeon general's report, the American Heart Association, the American Cancer Society, and virtually every legitimate study on human nutrition of the past 25 years. In fact, it will epitomize these recommendations. And luscious fruits, colorful vegetables, hearty whole grains, and legumes satisfy hunger while they discourage cravings. With a loving attitude and these foods as the staples in your kitchen, you can eat all you want because you will want just what you need. Weight loss and maintenance will proceed spontaneously without undue attention. You can stop watching your weight and start seeing the beauty that is in and around you. In this way, Love works in you to make your life better and through you to make your world better.

There's an old maxim that says, "He who lives for himself alone lives for the meanest mortal known." Those who eat for themselves alone are in something of the same category. That's one reason why diets consistently fail. Instead of bringing you into the stream of life, they set you apart from it—off somewhere with your blender and your portion scale and your food diary. In loving yourself thin, however, you'll recognize that you are not only a part of life, you are a vital part of it. Love has a vested interest in getting you out of your food rut because you will be vastly more loving when you are.

Is this going to be complicated? No, it's deceptively simple. Will it be easy? Not all the time, but living this way is, at its toughest, easier than trying to convince yourself that the half-gallon of ice cream in your shopping cart is for the family, when you know that your husband is out of town and both your kids are allergic to it. Probably the most difficult thing you'll have to grapple with is giving up the fight. You may feel as if you've gone AWOL (absent without leave), but believe me: With Love as your commander-in-chief, you'll be honorably discharged from active combat. You'll be able to harmonize an inner awareness of Love with loving outward actions—food choices included.

This harmony is essential for durable change, whether you want to overcome chronic binge eating, do away with an annoying 10 pounds, stop dieting for the first time since puberty, or simply eat a little more healthfully than you do now. Life without the dual plagues of compulsive eating and fanatical weight control is precious indeed. Health of body and peace of mind are also priceless commodities. To help you toward these, love yourself to a new relationship with food; love yourself to a new appreciation for yourself and your body; and love yourself thin instead of forcing yourself there.

ONE
Food as a Fix

I WAS A FAT LITTLE GIRL IN A FAT-PHOBIC FAMILY. There was always a diet for me taped to the refrigerator and I only got a milk shake when I was sick. Years later, I had a cold and my boyfriend brought me a French vanilla shake. I married him. You see, my father had been a physician who had gradually turned his practice from ear, nose, and throat to fat, flab, and cellulite. My mother managed "reducing salons" with adipose-jiggling machines and the promise of effortless weight loss. I knew early on that my plumpness was not pleasing and that I was bad for business.

It wasn't that I didn't want to be good and stick to my diet. I knew that there were starving children who didn't even have grapefruit and broiled halibut, but the notion of restricting what I ate was terrifying. It meant giving up the sublime security that came from an illicit cookie or bowl of ice cream. When I was eating, I felt safe, content, and loved. Once the food was gone, so was the feeling. I needed food to sustain life like everybody else, but I also needed it to face life. I didn't know it then, but I was hooked. Food was my fix.

When I was 13, I discovered the flip side of my addiction: the high of being thin. I'd had a severe case of measles and wasn't able to eat for a couple of weeks. Once I got out of bed, I weighed myself: 111 pounds. I had bones. They were wonderful. I was wonderful. I bought a gorgeous green satin dress with puffy sleeves and a dropped waist and a flippy little skirt. I was awed by my own reflection in the mirror. Although only 5 feet 5 inches, I looked to myself like the models in the teen magazines. I could have died in peace at that moment: I was finally okay.

I never got to go anywhere in that green satin dress, though. Within a month I was back to 140 pounds and felt for the first time "pitiful and incomprehensible demoralization." That's the phrase the book *Alcoholics Anonymous* uses to describe the state of an alcoholic who had once gained some control and then lost it again. I never drank, but the phrase fit.

I didn't realize then that control for me, just as for an alcoholic, wasn't the point. I was sick when it came to food, and I could no more control my eating than I could control the healing of a broken leg. That's why all my stalwart attempts at managing my eating ended as dismal failures.

One of these came in young adulthood with a popular commercial weight-loss system. I followed the recommended diet with religious fervor, refusing to alter it in any way. Even after I reached my goal weight of 120, I stayed on the diet until I weighed in one Saturday morning at 98 pounds. That did it: I had broken the thin barrier. I was cured. I bought a pound of roasted cashews, ate them all on the bus ride home, and gained 20 pounds in 40 days. "Pitiful and incomprehensible demoralization" combined with such hatred for my inflated body that I refused to be seen by anyone who knew me. I quit my job and moved to Chicago where I planned to hide, diet, and return at some future date in triumphant thinness.

While in Chicago, I learned to fast, perfecting 14-day stints on water only and doing several short juice fasts as well. My physical self shrunk obediently every time, but I was so ravenous after each of these "Gandhian" intervals that I ate enough to go back home in 1½ years with nearly 60 more pounds to my credit. After that, I stayed away from scales.

It took months for my ability to diet to resurface. It was inspired by my boyfriend's taking off for the West Coast, maybe to come back, maybe not. Hurt and anger mobilized my resolve: I would get thin and beautiful and show him what he'd left behind. I lost weight and he proposed, but neither of us realized that I was a food addict, a fact that the size of my body could not alter.

The facade started to crack with little weight gains here and there. They were frightening, and I felt I couldn't trust myself around a refrigerator while subject to any of the ordinary pressures of life—work, my roommate, my cat ... The answer: fat farms! I took a week in Texas the first time, then two in

Florida. It was becoming an expensive habit, so I started checking myself in at nice local hotels to diet or fast and use their health club facilities. It worked well for a while, but as I needed to go more frequently, cost again became an issue.

I looked for cheaper and cheaper hotels. The last one was a past-its-prime hostelry in the middle of town. The room cost $5. It had a phone book minus the Yellow Pages and a Gideon Bible lacking most of the New Testament. The carpet had been burned in spots by a careless smoker and the television was chained to the wall. "I'm in a bona fide flophouse," I told myself. "This is skid row and I've made my way here with a fork." I cried most of the night because I knew I had become the equivalent of a gutter drunk, but if I told anyone that, they'd laugh and tell me to go on a diet.

I knew that I was sick and that sick people are supposed to see physicians. I was wary of diet doctors; I had tried appetite-suppressing shots and pills before and got more wired than wiry. This time I decided to seek the services of a general practitioner who suggested testing me for hypoglycemia (low blood sugar). I took some comfort in the prospect of a genuine diagnosis, especially since so many of the hypoglycemic symptoms sounded like mine: a craving for food, especially sweets, and a gripping panic when deprived of food for a long period, accompanied with depression, irritability, and moodiness.

I was scheduled for a 6-hour glucose-tolerance test, a grueling ordeal of breaking a 12-hour fast with a bottle of pure glucose and having blood drawn seven times in the next 6 hours while taking in no other food. By the end of the test, I thought I was going to die: I was nervous, shaky, and dizzy and would have sold my soul for a turnip. I went straight from the hospital to a convenience store and bought two candy bars, a bag of chips, an ice cream bar, and a diet soda. When the test results turned out to be normal, I was sure that there had been a mistake. I convinced the doctor to arrange for me to be tested whenever I experienced the shakes and lightheadedness that I felt signaled hypoglycemia. I rushed to the lab during a particularly severe episode, expecting to find my blood sugar at some subterranean level. It was normal.

After a half-dozen such forays, I had to accept that the symptoms I was experiencing were not from hypoglycemia. They were withdrawal. When I didn't have that comforting sense of fullness, the friendly and accomplished young woman that I often seemed to be gave way to the frightened child who had found comfort in soft white bread and sweet sandwich cookies.

Seeing that kind of emotional connection to food, my next step was to enter counseling. The psychologists I saw pointed out numerous reasons why I ate the way I did. The list was impressive.

1. I'd had a digestive disorder as an infant, so I carried with me a primal fear of starvation.

2. My parents' professions had set me up for an eating disorder. My staying overweight was an unconscious ploy to demand their unconditional love.

3. Since I had been a fat child, I had a greater number of fat cells than people who had never been heavy or who had gained weight in adulthood and simply enlarged the fat cells they already had. All those greedy lipid cells were crying out to be fed.

4. I had, according to one unconventional therapist, died of hunger in a former incarnation and was trying to make up for it in this one.

I was grateful to learn all these fascinating hypotheses about my behavior. Unfortunately, being so enlightened didn't change a thing. My physicians had no remedy for my body and my therapists had none for my mind, although I was in need on both counts. The solution, if there was to be one, had to come in another way. And it did. I didn't outgrow my food addiction, I don't have any more willpower than I ever did, and I haven't had broiled halibut in more than 25 years. Nevertheless, I didn't eat for a fix today and I didn't obsess over the size and shape of my body. As a practicing food addict, I was helpless, but I was never hopeless. Neither are you.

PATTERNS

YOU MAY EAT FOR A FIX IN MANY OF THE WAYS THAT I DID. The pattern may have started early in life or when you got married or after you were divorced. You may trace it to a pregnancy or the loss of someone you loved, or it may have come upon you subtly and gradually. You may eat enormous meals or snack all day and not even remember when you had your last real breakfast, lunch, or dinner. You may only eat unreasonably when it comes to chocolates or other sugary foods or salty, crunchy snacks. Perhaps you eat sparingly around people and binge on the sly so no one can understand why you don't lose weight. ("She eats like a bird," you've heard them say, "but she's as big as a horse.")

On the other hand, you may be enviably slim and only you know that you stay that way by throwing up every day or that your preoccupation with fitness long ago shifted from a healthy habit to a tyrannical compulsion. You could be eating quite reasonably and looking fine but you feel fat, berate yourself, and want to live in a body that your heredity didn't provide. Maybe you're so devastated by the addiction that you avoid people as much as you can and hardly bother to wash the one outfit that you can still wear. More likely, though, you seem to function flawlessly and keep on top of everything, except for a little problem with eating. It's also possible that you don't have a serious problem with food or your body image at all, but it's been six months since your doctor told you to make some changes in your diet to lower your cholesterol or your blood pressure and you haven't been able to do it to save your life.

Whatever category you belong to, you've probably said, "I guess I just like food too much." Well, of course you like food. Everybody does. We're supposed to like it so much that we eat it as long as we live and live as long as we can. That's nature's way. It's only when food seems to choose us instead of our choosing it that something is wrong. Any time we stuff ourselves, starve ourselves, or eat something we know to be harmful, we're mistreating ourselves in ways that we don't deserve. When we do any of these things repeatedly, we establish a self-destructive and self-defeating pattern. When we want to stop but can't, we're addicted.

Some would argue with that terminology. They would say that food is not a drug that is universally addictive like heroin or even selectively addictive like alcohol. They might argue that food can cause, at worst, a behavioral addiction. The phenomenon of craving, however, exists in food addiction as in any other kind of addiction. It was powerful enough to send me out on foot at midnight in search of caramels. I once craved food so strongly that I took leftover cake from an office wastebasket, brushed off the cigarette ashes, and ate all but the cardboard plate.

I also know that food can be the object of addiction because I see others and myself recovering by using spiritual principles of transformation. The spiritual approach is also without equal in helping people addicted to other substances and practices. The only real difference in getting over a food addiction as opposed to an addiction to alcohol or cocaine is one of abstemiousness versus abstinence. Alcoholics stop drinking alcohol. Drug addicts stop using mood-altering drugs. Food addicts can't give up eating, but we can stop eating for a fix. Recovery is a delicate balance somewhere between the binge and the diet. That's where we abandon the struggle and find sanity and peace of mind.

The dictionary defines recovery as "to get back." For me, it has meant getting back some surprising things. One of them is my youth. I spent so much of my earlier life in the disease that even though I'm nearing 50, I delight in looking and feeling younger than I am. I'm able to use the nutritional knowledge that I had in abundance (food addicts love learning about food) but could never apply. Those physicians and counselors that I dismissed as worthless can be helpful now when I consult them for guidance instead of expecting them to provide me with the transformation that had to come from within. I've even gotten back the joy of eating. What I did before was drugging, and it was seldom pleasant to my stomach or my conscience. Eating is a pleasure today—that's how it should be. But it's a peripheral pleasure, not the center of my world. And this is not some new, post-diet euphoria: It has been like this for me, one day following another, for 15 years.

I once hated the way that I ate but couldn't change it. The difference started when I gave up willpower for the power of Love—Love for myself and from myself, for others and from them, and grounded in the Love that is also power. I'm comfortable calling that God. You can call it whatever you like. It has, by any name, provided an answer where there seemed to be none, and a life beyond the fix that's filled with hope and humor and expectation. Tapping that power is essential for addicts to live again, and my hunch is that some of that same power is needed for almost anyone to make major lifestyle changes that last. If you do not believe in miracles, or if you think that they don't happen anymore, just come to my house for dinner.

Some Things That Food Addicts May Do

- Hide food
- Sneak food

- Go on diets, usually on Mondays
- Make promises, vows, and deals with themselves, others, and God about eating less and losing weight
- Lie to themselves, others, and God
- Avoid scales or weigh themselves compulsively
- Dissociate from their bodies—live from the neck up
- Put off living (shopping, swimming, vacationing, making love) until weight is lost
- Detest physical exercise or become addicted to exercise (but may still detest it)
- Feel unattractive or conditionally attractive based upon a scale number or clothing size
- Hate fat people (or thin people)
- Have special binge foods as drugs of choice (chocolate, sweets, and salty snacks are favorites) but could binge on almost anything in a pinch
- Eat others' leftovers, unthawed frozen foods, or nonfoods (such as wrappers from muffins, used tea bags, or chewing gum)
- Vomit after a binge or even after a moderate meal or snack (known as bulimia)
- Diet successfully for a time, then gain back as much as or more weight than was lost (the ability to diet eventually ceases altogether)
- Fast at times relatively easily, finding it less trying to eat nothing than to eat moderately
- Feed other people, especially when depriving themselves
- Cook and bake—though in later stages of the disease, these may fall aside in favor of ready-made, instant-gratification items
- Please people, be "sweet"
- Deal inappropriately with anger, either denying ("stuffing") it or having attacks of rage, usually toward someone powerless such as a child or pet
- Switch compulsions, such as giving up food for a time and becoming addicted to drugs (like diet pills), relationships, or spending

Some Things That Food Addicts May Think

- This diet/pill/doctor will be the one that works.
- I ate too much (or gained weight), so I'm a bad person.
- No one else eats like I do.
- If you really knew me, you wouldn't like me.
- I'm fat and disgusting.
- I broke my diet, so I'm a failure.
- I ate two extra peas. That means I've blown it and have to eat half a gallon of ice cream.
- I've lost weight now and so life is supposed to be perfect.
- I've lost weight now, so I'm cured.
- This time I'll just have a little bit.
- I'll get back on my diet tomorrow.
- Eating will make me feel better.
- I have to eat something to get through this tragedy/term paper/telephone call.
- When I lose weight, I'll be beautiful.
- When I lose weight, my husband/wife/lover will love me (or, I'll get a husband/wife/lover).
- When I lose weight, my mother/father/other significant person will love and accept me (even if they're dead).
- When I lose weight, I'll do everything I ever wanted to do.
- I feel fat (in response to being full, depressed, premenstrual, or constipated, but also in response to rejection, disappointment, or presumed failure).
- If I eat while I read, it won't count (the same goes for food sampled during cooking).
- I deserve a treat (euphemism for extra food), or I deserve to be punished (food can do that, too).

Some Things That People Say to Food Addicts (That Don't Help at All)

- Use a little willpower.
- Push yourself away from the table.
- I've got this great diet for you.
- Just eat less.
- How could you let yourself get this way?
- I need to be perfectly honest with you … (followed by almost anything).
- You have such a pretty face.
- I remember when you wore a size 6 (or 8 or 10 or 14).
- Your sister/brother/friend trimmed down so nicely.
- I'll come over at 6:00 tomorrow and we'll jog.
- Come on. You'll have to shape up if you want to attract the ladies (or men).
- I don't know how to tell you this, but do you realize that you have a weight problem?
- You really look perfectly fine … well, except you could lose a few pounds.
- You're too old to change how you eat (or, you're too young not to).
- I'm only concerned about your health.
- You know, gluttony is a sin.
- Take one of these pills whenever you get hungry.
- Beauty is only skin deep anyhow.
- Do what I did and put a sign on your refrigerator that says, "Oink!"
- You can have just one (or, a little won't hurt this once).
- I made this especially for you.
- You'd feel so much better about yourself if you lost a little weight.
- I clipped out this article about how being overweight shortens life expectancy.
- I lost five pounds taking these great vitamins—in fact, I'm selling them.
- You just need to get a hold of yourself (with or without an addendum about how much of oneself there is to get hold of).

TWO
The Body and the Spirit

LIKE STEPCHILDREN IN FAIRY TALES, OUR BODIES GET BLAMED FOR A LOT. When we criticize them, we put ourselves down, too. If you've ever said, "I hate my thighs," or "I used to be pretty but now I'm a wreck," or "Look at this fat—I'm really disgusting!" you've been your own evil stepmother.

Your weight may be a problem, but it isn't *the* problem. It's a symptom—usually a symptom of an unhealthy or unloving relationship with food. You can be rid of the symptom while the real problem flourishes. Getting thin is not a cure. Any size 4 person with bulimia can attest to that. Nevertheless, if you deal with the cause of the overweight, your body will reflect a wellness, a balance, and a beauty that go far beyond how you look in a pair of shorts.

INNER MALAISE = DESTRUCTIVE EATING = OVERWEIGHT

There's a continuum here. It starts with what I'm calling inner malaise. That's a catchall term to cover fear and discontent, stress and impaired self-image, emotional leftovers from childhood, or anything else that stands between us and our being at peace with ourselves and our world. Inner malaise can lead to a variety of inappropriate or self-destructive behaviors. Destructive eating is the one we're concerned with. It generally shows up as extra weight.

Traditionally, we've gone after the obvious: the weight. And why not? We can see it. We can even weigh it, for heaven's sake. But when it's gone (via diets, exercise, pills, you name it), the inner malaise can still be active, resulting in further destructive eating. In fact, as long as the inner malaise goes unchecked, even dieting is destructive eating (or destructive noneating). It will eventually lead to gaining back the lost weight, or to some variation on the theme, such as bulimia.

This is not to say that there are no physical reasons for overweight: There are several. Scientists have found evidence that low levels of a hormone called leptin may cause some men and women—perhaps 10 percent of overweight people—to carry extra weight. And for some people with food and weight problems, refined sugars and greasy, salty snacks seem to cause an addictive reaction that leads to overeating. Too much fat in your diet can result in too much fat on your body, and lack of exercise can lower your metabolic rate, encouraging fat storage.

Dieting itself is also a factor. The deprivation of dieting can cause a physical and emotional backlash that Neal Barnard, M.D., calls the restrained eater phenomenon. He writes in his book *The Power of Your Plate*, "The body cannot distinguish dieting from starvation....We are automatically driven to gorge ourselves in anticipation of recurrent famine."

Another problem with dieting is that it is generally earmarked by taste deprivation. According to ancient Indian teachings, we need to experience the full spectrum of taste in order to feel satisfied. The typical Westerner eats foods that are primarily sweet and salty, largely depriving the taste buds of sour, bitter, pungent (spicy), and astringent sensations. (Astringent refers to the clean and slightly dry taste of foods like beans, apples, and cabbage.) Dieters restrict themselves even further. When we don't get all six tastes each day—and preferably at each full meal—we feel that something is missing. We think that we need second helpings or dessert or cafeteria-style evenings of one snack after another. One solution to taste deprivation is to include a bit of the Indian condiment chutney, made from a variety of fruits and spices, with every meal. Another is to eat adequately of a wide variety of real foods and not live in mortal terror of their caloric content.

Knowing about the various physical reasons that may underlie an off-kilter relationship with food is obviously quite different than doing something about them. What is it that keeps so many people from doing what they know would bring them what they want? For a great many people—and only you can decide if you're one of them—inner malaise blocks their attempts to put into practice the good things they already know about nutrition and a healthy lifestyle.

Some people have realized that attacking the weight is a hopeless maneuver, and they have proposed alternative plans of action that focus on the second part of the equation: the eating itself. Their strategy is generally behavior modification—techniques such as taking small bites and putting the fork down between them, or forgoing the fork altogether and giving chopsticks a try. The idea behind these techniques is to shut out old habits with new ones, like not eating alone or not eating after 7:00 P.M. These can be positive practices, but most of the time they fail over the long haul. Why? They fail because our actions ultimately grow out of ourselves. Unless we change, our actions are not likely to change in any long-term way.

On the other hand, when the inner malaise itself is addressed, both harmful eating patterns and their resultant overweight lose their source and sustenance. Tiny miracles transpire one by one. We take those smaller bites. We aren't hanging on to the fork as if it were a life preserver. Breathing gets easier. Clothes get looser. And although we never asked for this one, life gets better. It has to, because it is being lived in a new and decidedly better way.

HEALING AT THE DESIRE LEVEL

WHEN HEALING COMES LIKE THIS, from within, it's healing at the desire level. It's no longer wanting a chocolate bar and settling for an orange; it's wanting the orange and relishing every bite of it. Of course, this does not mean that there will never again be food choices to make. There are healthful and unhealthful food choices just as there are healthful and unhealthful life choices. Only by dealing with the inner malaise, though, are we able to truly make choices about what we eat. Otherwise, the choices are made for us, and we usually regret them.

When we turn to unhealthful or excessive food (or any other damaging substance or practice) in order to feel better, it's because something is missing in our lives. Although it seems that what we lack is outside ourselves—the right job, the right mate, the right body, the right memories—the emptiness is core-deep. To make satisfying, lasting changes in how we nourish our bodies, we must learn to get some vital nourishment from within. We do that by connecting with our spiritual selves, by making practical contact with the Divine, whatever we perceive that to be.

If you can get past the binge/diet syndrome by some other means, terrific. I couldn't. I had stressed my resolve and my willpower until, like overworked peasants, they chose to revolt. That insidious urge to smooth life's rough edges with a nibble that could turn into a nightmare would overtake me just when I was convinced that I had everything under control. My intelligence and good intentions were of no more use than lighting fixtures in a house with no wiring. I needed power and I didn't have it. I needed to tap into a Higher Power, one that would always be there.

It was such a strange notion. My problem had seemed so physical. I ate quantities of physical food and it showed quantitatively on my physical body, yet paradoxically, the answer to my problem was spiritual. It didn't make sense to me at first, and it may not make sense to you until you realize that, as human beings, we are like icebergs. What people see, our physical selves, is only the tip of who we are. There's a lot more beneath the surface. We're splendid beings with complex emotions and intellects, and underlying our hearts, minds, and bodies is a spiritual essence. It is uniquely ours, yet it connects us to every living thing. It connects us to life itself.

The part of you that shows, your body, is important because it is a part of you and you are important. You can think of your body as the vehicle by which you journey through this life, as your radio receiver for picking up the signals of the outside world, or as an instrument in an orchestra, allowing you to play your music for the rest of us. A symphony needs French horns and oboes, cellos and violins, tinkling little triangles and booming bass drums. You might even be a grand piano.

Abusing food can interfere with your ability to appreciate your special physical self. In an all-out binge, it's necessary to, in effect, cut off diplomatic relations between the body and the mind. Since it's a rare person who consciously wants to be miserable, most people who binge separate their conscious (thinking) selves from their sensory (physical) selves by reading, working, driving, or watching television while they eat. They may absentmindedly grab snacks throughout the day or tastes while cooking a meal. Swearing off the distractions that remove you from the present moment may seem like the antidote, but it isn't. If you have the need to binge, you will find a way to shut off your mind—with all its "shoulds" and "oughts" and "know betters"—and go for the food.

The need to binge is a spiritual hunger. It can only be assuaged with spiritual food. Did you know that koala bears eat nothing but eucalyptus leaves? The soul is something like that. It can only be nourished by Love. You see, all genuine love is good—love from your family, your friends, even your companion animals—but the kind that you need for this purpose can't be filtered through anyone else. It has to be from the source: Love that is within you so you don't have to look for it, that is already yours so you don't have to earn it, that can't stop loving so you needn't worry about losing it. Once you realize that this Love exists, that it's available to you with no questions asked, you'll be eager to put into practice the principles that you will learn in this book. The first are these.

1. Accept that your food problem is serious, that you can't deal with it on your own.

2. Open your mind to the idea that a Higher Power can help.

3. Allow that Power—call it Love, call it God, call it whatever feels absolutely right to you—to work some wonders in your life.

If you're familiar with the Twelve Steps of Alcoholics Anonymous, adopted by Overeaters Anonymous, Gamblers Anonymous, Codependents Anonymous, and numerous other groups, you'll recognize these three concepts as an interpretation of the first three steps. People in the anonymous programs sometimes abbreviate these steps as, "I can't, God can, I'll let Him (or Her or It)." However worded, this formula is common to men and women of all ages and cultures who have built or rebuilt their lives on a spiritual basis, letting go of old ways that didn't work and inviting in something that does.

A LIFETIME ADVENTURE

SPIRITUALIZING YOUR THOUGHTS AND ATTITUDES is an adventure that can last a lifetime. To instigate the process, particularly as it affects your eating, take the following actions today and every day for the next month.

1. Each morning before your feet touch the floor, ask your Higher Power to help you eat reasonably that day and say thank you at night even if your eating didn't seem perfect.

2. When you get to a mirror to wash your face or shave, look yourself in the eye and say, "I love you just the way you are." You don't have to believe it yet, just do it.

3. Read over the "Revolutionary Concepts" (see page 24) every morning and evening.

4. Spend some quiet time by yourself every single day—at least 10 minutes' worth. If you have to take this time in the bathtub to get privacy, fine. During this quiet, read over the first three of the Twelve Steps (see page 243) and think about them. Do you really believe that you're powerless over your addiction or is there something else you'd like to try? Can you contemplate the possibility that a Higher Power could help? Can you consider making a decision to put that Higher Power in charge of your will and your life? (Writing your thoughts on this in a journal isn't required, but it can be helpful. There's room at the end of this book if you want to get started.)

5. Do not diet. Think instead in terms of not eating for a fix one day at a time. Get three reasonable meals every day (or as many reasonable meals as you and your health care providers have established as ideal for your particular situation). Before each meal (and before each planned snack if you have them), ask your Higher Power to help you eat wisely. If you want to eat at other times, converse with your Higher Power. If you're really hungry, have a piece of fruit. Eat it slowly. Enjoy it.

6. Do two nice things for yourself today—one that you think you should do (make the bed, floss your teeth, swim laps) and one that's just for fun (take a bubble bath, rent a video, call a friend). Don't be surprised if it's easier to enjoy the work than the play.

7. Enlist some support. At the very least, read this book with a friend and then help each other along. You'll do yourself a far greater favor if you hook up with a support group already organized that uses proven principles to help food addicts recover. I recommend Overeaters Anonymous (OA). This group will teach you how to incorporate the Twelve Steps into your life while providing an unparalleled support system of people who understand. OA meetings are in every major city and most smaller ones, and there is no charge for membership. (For more information on the organization, see page 242.)

If you're feeling overwhelmed by all this, relax. You're not in a competition and you don't have to pass a quiz. Many of these ideas may be new to you. Give yourself time to let them settle—you may want to read this chapter more than once before you go further. You're embarking on a transformational journey. That's no small thing. It's certainly understandable if you're feeling some trepidation. There is a lot at stake here. Old patterns of doing things are going to be replaced. They don't want to get fired.

While you're making layoffs, you may also want to consider trading any old images of a punishing, wrathful deity for a Higher Power that loves you no matter what. You'll need one that isn't just interested in great, cosmic events but one that is interested in you and in seeing you out of your food addiction. The image that I like is of God as the sun, shining upon each and every one of us with our own personal beam, keeping us safe and warm. You can use any image that speaks to you. Just get used to being loved unconditionally. Before long, you'll be loving yourself unconditionally, too. (Unconditional, you know, includes thighs.)

You are not only lovable but also, whether you realize it or not, spiritual. Do not think for an instant that because the solution to food addiction is spiritual, food addicts themselves somehow aren't. In the midst of a binge, anyone's spirituality is on temporary hold, but your inherent spiritual identity persists. Being overweight or in some other way obsessed with food or with your body does not negate that identity.

All the inner growth you've done up to this point counts, too. Only you and God know how far you've had to come to get here, to the point where you can look honestly at yourself and what you are eating. Give yourself some credit and resist the urge to compare yourself to anyone else. Many people have never had a serious problem with food. Others have overcome food addictions while you were growing through something else. All that matters now is that you've suffered with this long enough. It's your turn to be free—body and spirit.

PHASE OUT FAT DAYS
• • • • • • • • • • • • • • • • • • •

Do you ever have fat days? On fat days you feel fat regardless of your size. These days can be precipitated by eating way too much, a little too much, or just what you think is too much. They can also be brought on by such seeming irrelevancies as having dirty hair or an argument with someone who's important in your life. Losing weight isn't a fully satisfactory response to fat days since they're so subjective. As an extreme but telling example, think of people with anorexia. I've visited some in hospitals who were painfully, even frighteningly, emaciated, yet who felt fat. For them, every day was a fat day, although they had actually been in danger of dying from lack of nourishment.

While anorexia is a psychiatric disorder that requires professional help, seeing the body in a distorted way is so common that it's generally accepted as the way things are. But what if instead of fat days you had poison-ivy days—days when you itched all over even though there was nothing organically wrong? It would seem like a problem, wouldn't it? Well, fat days are a problem, too, because they're days on which you tend to love yourself less than you deserve. You are lovable every day. You can't force yourself to believe that, but you can allow the possibility that it is true to enter your world view. Allowing for such possibilities is a spiritual activity because it happens deep within you.

A long time ago a friend said to me, "When I'm 150 pounds going up, I'm the fattest, ugliest person on Earth, but when I'm 150 coming down, I'm absolutely beautiful." In the years since she made that statement, my friend has done a lot of inner work to realize that she's beautiful all the time. It so happens that she hasn't had an eating binge in 20 years, and the notion of "going up" and "coming down" primarily affects her today as it relates to elevators and airplane trips.

Spiritual recovery means more than an end to eating for a fix. It also implies befriending your body. You don't wait to do that until after you've reached some arbitrary goal weight. You do it today, the first day that you put your food choices in the hands of a loving Higher Power. The imaging ability of the mind that can be twisted to give you fat days can be uplifted to give you attractive and healthy days. As these days go by, your physical body will catch up with your mental image. Since the body is subject to physical laws, it will take some time for its form to change, but the time it takes for you to be happy and to have an attractive, healthy day is no time at all.

REVOLUTIONARY CONCEPTS

THESE REVOLUTIONARY CONCEPTS AREN'T FOR TAKING OVER EMBASSIES, they're the beginner's basics for revolutionizing your relationship with your body and how you feed it. Read them over every morning and evening for 30 days, paying particular attention to those with which you may feel uncomfortable. It's possible that those won't apply to you at all, but it's more likely that they're precisely the ones that can mean the most in your recovery.

- You are acceptable right now, regardless of what you ate yesterday or what the scale has to say about you.
- Abusing food is a sign of internal imbalance, and overcoming it is largely an inside job.
- Food addiction is serious and, like other addictions, progressive. Few genuine addicts have ever recovered without a spiritual basis.
- Your spirituality is personal. You don't have to take on someone else's brand.
- You are a spiritual being living in a physical body. Your body is an integral part of the totality that is you.
- Your body is not an independent entity; it reflects what is going on inside you—emotionally, mentally, and spiritually.
- It's okay to feel beautiful right now. If you wait until you're thin to feel beautiful, you may never get there.
- If you don't eat for a fix today, that long string of tomorrows that seems so foreboding will take care of itself.
- Your body is not your enemy. You and your body are in this together. When you do something nice for your body, you're doing something nice for yourself.

- Having a food addiction does not make you a bad person. Both medicine and psychology recognize addiction as an illness, not a moral issue.
- You don't have to be perfect to get well, and it's even all right to be a little bit scared.
- Ideas that you're not sure of can be tried out, like taking a car on a test drive. If, for example, the thought of a spiritual solution to your food problem doesn't seem logical, you can consider it a possibility, a working hypothesis.

THREE
Getting to Point Zero

RACE IS ONLY FAIR IF EVERY CONTESTANT STARTS AT THE STARTING LINE. If life were a race, though, some of us would have to run a veritable marathon just to get to the place where everyone else seems fresh and rested, eager to take off. I call that place Point Zero. At Point Zero, you're free, unencumbered, and your chances for winning are as good as anybody's. Eating for a fix, however, can keep you from getting there.

Healthy people meet every new day, every new dilemma, every new project from the level ground of Point Zero. Because they like themselves, they're comfortable with life and aren't likely to become addicted to anything. They're not perfect and don't need to be, but they're at home in their own skins and in the world around them. When they have difficulties, they're able to get the help they need and use the help they get, whether it comes from friends, family, professionals, or their own inner resources. They rebound well from adversity and although they may lose many things in life, hope won't be one of them. At Point Zero, there is always hope, spirited challenge, and limitless potential.

Addictive behavior keeps Point Zero elusive. Food addicts now in recovery have described it in these ways.

I felt like I was in an invisible box and couldn't get out. People kept offering me advice and ideas that I couldn't use because I couldn't get out of the box to try them. I see now that I'd built the box myself and that I'd built it with a tight-fitting lid.

There was one awful thing in my life: the way I ate. I was really angry that I couldn't do anything about it since I seemed to be so good at everything else. It seemed like a terrible blight to me, a stigma.

My life looked great: I was busy all the time. But when I was alone, something always seemed to be missing. I was experiencing a quiet desperation. I acted happy, you know, "jolly," but I was so sad.

As you can see from the diagram on page 28, Point Zero is sort of an alchemical crossroads at which the old baggage of subzero attitudes and actions is turned into golden qualities. Obsessive eating no longer fits. You accept life on life's terms. You're a participant in it instead of a spectator. Fear is transmuted into safe, healing, unconditional love. It provides the foundation for the best possible relationships with yourself, other people, and the myriad things that make up your life, your work, your interests, your finances, your food. When you clear away what stands between you and Point Zero, you will be able to tap into that Love, which has always been available, more easily than ever before. Once you do, you'll find yourself showing up when life is passing the good stuff your way, and when circumstances aren't the best, you won't be brought down so far with them.

The fear-motivated thought and action patterns you see on the diagram beneath the zero point lead away from self-love and self-care. It doesn't make you a bad person to be acquainted with those patterns; they are simply thoughts and actions that don't work to bring you what you want in life. They worked at one time or you wouldn't have developed them. They were protection mechanisms that were once useful but have come to do more harm than good, like an old pair of glasses that used to help you see better but now make everything a blur. It's time for a new prescription.

Using food or extra weight as a buffer between yourself and life is one way to keep old patterns intact and stay negative, in the red, below Point Zero. This does not mean that because you and I have histories of misusing food

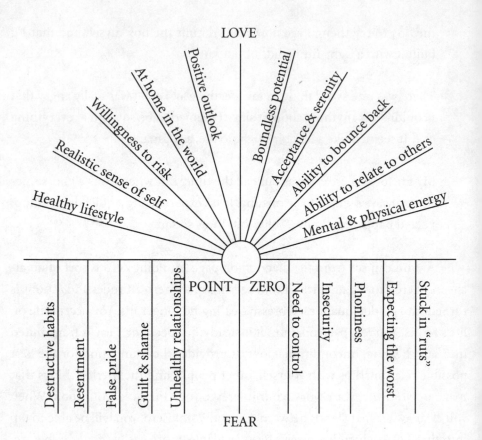

that we are, or ever were, less valuable than the next person. The fact that we're alive makes us remarkable. Besides, you can come from a respected family and be highly intelligent, well-educated, and gainfully employed but still feel subzero inside.

It may manifest as feeling out of place much of the time or as if you're somehow different from other people. You may be tired of trying to catch up to some invisible goal or meet some impossible standard. You may recognize as your own some of the subzero thinking patterns in "A Mental Makeover" on page 49. However much or little you relate to these examples, if you're still using food in a way that you're uncomfortable with (or if you're not right now but are afraid you will again), there is some distance between you and the freedom you'll find at Point Zero.

Your mission, then, is to get to Point Zero from wherever you're starting. In one sense, there isn't far to go—only about 12 inches, the distance from your head to your heart. In terms of consciousness, however, this may be the most meaningful journey you've ever taken. You won't make it to Point Zero alone or by sheer effort or willpower. You need to resign yourself to being the passenger on this trip: Love (God, a Higher Power) will do the driving. You only need to get in the car. Your willingness to do that uses your will to the best advantage.

You started on the trek to Point Zero in the preceding chapter when you came to grips with the fact that you can't handle your food problem by yourself, when you allowed yourself to believe that a Higher Power could make the difference, and you decided to let that loving Power be in charge of things. You will reach Point Zero as you clean up the past and learn to live fearlessly and productively in the present. There are five things you must do.

1. Become more honest than you've ever been
2. Postpone eating for a fix
3. Sit with your feelings
4. Make peace with the past and with people
5. Expand your comfort zone

Underlying all of these are spiritual verities that have shown themselves over time to make people's lives better. Because truth is well-told in fable, I will introduce each one of the five ways for getting to Point Zero with a story.

BECOME MORE HONEST

There was once a shaman whose fame for miraculous healings spread far and wide. The people of his country were astounded by the miracles he performed and discoursed among themselves about how he accomplished them. "He becomes as tiny as a gnat," one suggested, "and goes into the sick body, sees what is wrong, and eats it away."

"No," argued another, "he becomes as tall as the sky and lifts
the sick person up to the gods. It is they who do the magic."

The shaman overheard this conversation and gently interrupted: "I am no larger or smaller than either of you, my friends.
And the healings that you see are not magic. I have simply spoken
the truth in earnestness for such a long time that my words cannot
be false. When I say that someone is well, he can be nothing else."

HONESTY IS NOT OPTIONAL if you want to live without a food problem. *The
Answer to Addiction*, a marvelous book by John Burns and three recovered alcoholics on overcoming addictions, explains it this way: "You connect with God
by means of the truth. And you connect with the truth by stopping lying."

Most of us don't think of ourselves as overt liars, but a solid commitment to
honesty is such a rarity that borderline dishonesty passes as acceptable and even
commendable. They're usually little things: A waiter forgets to charge for dessert
and the customer ignores it, or a six-year-old is passed off as five to get free admission into a theme park or a free ride on the bus. The individual incidents don't
amount to much, but they reflect a pervasive lack of regard for honesty in general. It wasn't long ago that "I give you my word" was as good as collateral, but
that's no longer the case. The result is that it takes a lot for people to trust one another. Even worse is the fact that we're often not sure we can trust ourselves.

Addiction breeds dishonesty, usually in subtle ways: "I really didn't eat
much dinner" (but you finished off all the leftovers), "I just didn't like anything
I tried on" (nothing fit), or "I think that I'll stay in tonight and get some work
done" (being home alone is a great way to binge in peace). To become more
honest, even if you believe that you're already as honest as you need to be, *The
Answer to Addiction* offers the following suggestions: "As a starter, stop lying to
yourself about your addicted condition.... Next, stop lying to get out of jams or
to smooth off the rough edges of life. Don't lie for the sake of peace; don't lie
when common sense invites you to do so; don't lie to cover up your past; don't
lie on job applications, expense accounts, or tax returns; don't lie to your boss;
don't lie to your husband or wife. Just don't lie. When you fail in this resolve (as
you will), admit it promptly. And don't indulge failure—that is, don't fail any
more than you have to."

An excellent place to initiate a commitment to honesty—although probably the most frightening—is as it concerns your eating. First, be honest with yourself about what you're putting into your mouth. Just because you eat something quickly and get rid of the wrapper, or because there isn't anyone else around, doesn't mean that you didn't eat it. Did you really have "a few potato chips" or was it a bag? If it was a bag, acknowledge that it was a bag. Denying reality doesn't change it, but dishonesty brings on dangerous rationalization: "I just had a few, so it won't make any difference if I have a few more."

While you're at it, it won't hurt to be honest about your weight. In a lot of ways, weight is a silly measurement of anything. It can fluctuate from day to day, and scales vary in their readings. But let's face it: You know just about how much you weigh. If you have to renew your driver's license, how awful would it be to tell the truth? Maybe it would be awful, but the perks you get back from telling the truth about everything are incredible. You deserve them.

Being truthful will hasten your progress toward freedom from the food fix more assuredly than any other single action. When your personal code of ethics includes both accepting the truth and speaking the truth, you'll see remarkable improvements in your life. Try this one: Commit yourself to a totally honest day and see how much easier it is to eat reasonably. I'll wager that you'll go to sleep that night with a particularly peaceful feeling.

Your experiment with expanded honesty will be helped tremendously if there are people around you that you can trust with honest confidences. These may be the ones who are closest to you, although sometimes it can be more difficult to be up front with significant others than with anyone else. Connecting with other food addicts who are committed to recovery, like those you'll come to know if you affiliate with Overeaters Anonymous, can be a real blessing in this regard. If nothing else, be sure that there is one other person in this world with whom you are willing to be absolutely honest, and share with him or her on a regular basis.

In time, dishonesty simply won't feel comfortable in any circumstance. This doesn't mean that you'll become harsh toward other people. "Honest to a fault" has been used to describe those who like to criticize. With honesty based on love, however, you'll be able to speak kindly and truthfully. You will also know when it's best to say nothing at all. This sort of intuition comes about as a result of your commitment to the truth. As that commitment grows, your true self—the one that is at Point Zero and is healthy, happy, and addiction-free—will start to emerge as well.

Honesty Exercises

- Drive within the speed limit, even when you're sure that you wouldn't get caught if you didn't.
- When you hear yourself putting yourself down ("I'm a slob," "I can't do anything right"), change the tape. Blanket put-downs of yourself or others do not reflect the truth.
- When you're wrong, say so.
- If a certain food has always been a problem for you (if one bite is too many and a thousand aren't enough), face it and leave that food alone.
- Abandon the cover-up, for yourself or others. If you forgot to return a call, say "I forgot." If your child didn't do her homework, don't help out with a subterfuge.
- Share with someone else exactly what you're eating, or at least write down honestly what you're eating and share it with yourself.
- Shop for food honestly. Do you really need to serve the scout troop your favorite kind of cookie? Are you truly expecting someone who dearly loves chocolates to just "drop by"?
- Be completely honest about your life and your feelings with one or more people you trust.
- Eat the same way when you're alone as when you're with people and vice versa.
- Be who you are wherever you are. If you have a chameleon suit, trade it in. Your beliefs, opinions, and preferences needn't be altered to fit one group or occasion and then another.
- When you find yourself exaggerating, bring the story down to size.
- Remember the important truth for food addicts: Alone, our prospects are grim, but there is a spiritual solution. Act on that truth.

POSTPONE EATING FOR A FIX

A severe storm destroyed all the huts in a small village. In the days that followed, the villagers were hard at work reconstructing their dwellings before the next rain. One man alone sat at the site where his hut had been, gathering no building materials and lifting no tools. "Why are you not building a shelter?" his neighbors queried. "The rains will come again soon."

The man was unmoved. "God took my house from me. He owes me another. I am waiting for God to build it." It was not long before the rains again poured down upon the village. The homeless man beat on the doors of his neighbors' houses, but the neighbors thought him lazy and would not let him in. He disappeared into the forest.

Some believe that he perished, but the wise tell their children how the man lost his senses in the woodland and lives there yet, wild and half-starved, his home the branches of a tree. "That," they warn the children, "is the best house you can expect if you refuse to give God a helping hand."

YOU CAN OFFER THAT HELPING HAND with your willingness to postpone the fix. When Love motivates your life, it will motivate your eating. A healthy relationship with food is one of the gifts that Love—genuine love for yourself as well as for others—will bring into your life. You accept this gift every time you refrain from using food for the wrong reasons.

It may seem paradoxical to suggest that you do so since the first step in recovery was the admission that you couldn't control your eating. That surrender, however, implied a transfer of power: You traded personal power for Love's power, God's power. Therefore, even if you think that you cannot possibly do it, you will be able to postpone eating for a fix. Recovering addicts of all stripes have used the "24-hours-at-a-time" method, which means that you only have to worry about not eating for a fix one day at a time. Deal with the 24-hour period you're living through right now, not the one tomorrow or a month from now. In dealing with other compulsions, it means not popping the first pill, placing the first bet, lighting the first cigarette, or in this case, swallowing the first inappropriate mouthful.

We're not able to say, "Starting this Monday, I'm going on 1,200 calories until I've lost 25 pounds." We've done that and sooner or later it has always backfired. What we are able to do is refrain from inappropriate eating today, just this day, from the time we awaken in the morning until we go to sleep at night. Neither yesterday nor tomorrow has any place in practicing a new way of life. It can only be done in the immediacy of the present.

As you work with spiritual ideas, your impulses to use food in unhealthy ways will diminish. Eventually, only in rare incidences will the urge to turn to food surface. When it does, you'll actually appreciate it as a signal that something isn't right inside. By then you'll have ample tools to use to get for yourself what you really need at that moment—probably some emotional or spiritual sustenance that can't be stored in a refrigerator. A supportive community, such as Overeaters Anonymous or something like it, can be invaluable at these times as well.

With your growing inner strength and the help of others, you can learn what you need from the feelings you're experiencing, long before they lead you to the kitchen or the deli. In the beginning, however, you may have the desire to eat inappropriately rather often. Inappropriate eating includes situations like these.

- It's 11:00 A.M. You're at the office. Your boss has told you to redo a report you've worked on all week. Lunch isn't for another hour, but as you look around, you think that you could eat this morning's mail, your Rolodex, and a fax machine.
- You're in bed with a cold. You just had a substantial lunch but it didn't taste like anything. Besides, there's nobody around to take care of you. A little something would really help, you know, a little sweet thing or a little salty thing.
- You've stopped smoking, but you miss the pleasant prolonging of dinner that a cigarette used to provide. Lately you've substituted with extra helpings and second desserts.
- There's no avoiding it: This is cleaning day. You had breakfast and you've descended on the bathrooms. You're fine on the basins and tubs, but then

come the floors. You hate doing floors. This seems like an ideal time for a snack.

- Your son's music lesson lasts an hour. It's not mealtime and you're not really hungry, but the only thing you can think of to do with the time between dropping him off and picking him up is to go somewhere for a bite.
- Your spouse brought in some cookies yesterday. They're the good ones. You know in your heart of hearts that eating one means eating the package, but you do it anyway.
- It's the middle of the night. You're up raiding the refrigerator and may not even remember how you got there. (Night eating can be a serious problem and professional help may be a valuable adjunct in the recovery process. Nevertheless, proven spiritual principles in tandem with group support have relieved all sorts of problem eaters, even the after-hours variety.)

Remember that as Love-powered living becomes a habit, trying situations can present themselves and you will almost never have the urge to respond to them with eating. When you do, the technique of postponement will prove invaluable. Start with a 24-hour solution. This is the day you're concerned about. You may need to shorten the time frame and be willing to put off the fix for 2 hours or 1 hour or for 15 minutes.

And what good does that do? Plenty. For one thing, if you've just finished a meal and want more, it may simply reflect physiological lag time. It takes about 20 minutes for the satiation center in your brain to register that you are full. When you allow that period of time to elapse, your desire to continue eating may abate and you will need to do nothing else. In addition, you can use that postponement time to get yourself centered. This is particularly important if you want to eat for emotional rather than physical reasons, even if you can't at the time tell one from the other.

Centering means finding that point of peace within yourself. It is there. It's there now, even if you're holding this book in your right hand and a doughnut in your left. The point of peace is with you when you're feeling angry, anxious, scared, or tired—and you *can* find it. Once there, you can easily connect with the power of Love that will do for you what food never could.

There are a variety of calming techniques such as relaxation and meditation to bring you to this state of mind (see Looking In, Reaching Out on page 52). Prayer or meditation at the time you want to open the refrigerator door can be of real help, provided that you truly want the help. Preventive prayer or making a routine of daily quiet time can fill empty places in advance so that you won't look to whatever is in the fridge to do it.

In addition to meditation and prayer, you can go from frantic to stable by engaging in any nondestructive activity that you enjoy. It's a smart move to make a list of the feel-good things you like to do, because if you wait until you want to eat everything that can't run faster than you, the only feel-good thing you'll be able to remember is eating. (You'll find a place at the end of this book to start such a list.) Photocopy your list and place a copy in several key spots: your bedside table, your desk at home and at the office, your car, and of course, somewhere in the kitchen. Your list will be your own. Mine is called Happy Stuff and looks like this.

1. Time with the people who matter most
2. Organizing some small space in my life, maybe a drawer or a closet
3. Comedy, even on TV
4. Brushing our cats
5. Going to a movie, especially those victory-of-the-human-spirit types
6. A hot bath
7. A circuit at the gym
8. Delicious music—the Pachelbel Canon, anything by Mozart
9. Stimulating conversation with someone whose company delights me
10. Making contact with nature: seeing a deer, feeding squirrels in the yard or pigeons in the park, or reading or writing in a pretty, natural spot

My list is actually longer than this. Happiness lists tend to grow as your awareness of the many pleasant things in life broadens. Obviously, the desire to eat inappropriately can strike when you aren't free to hop in the bathtub or take a book to the woods. Then you need immediate postponement techniques that also connect you with your spiritual source. Here are some examples.

- Read a paragraph or two of something helpful.
- Call someone you know to be supportive of your desire to eat rationally.
- Change your environment, even for a few minutes, like using your coffee break to get outside, walk around a little, breathe some fresher air.
- Write down how you're feeling and you may be surprised by what comes out; putting emotions and confusions down in black and white can be both revealing and freeing (you may think of it as praying on paper). There is room at the end of the book for this, too.
- Get by yourself, even it it's in the washroom, for a brief quiet time.
- Ask your Higher Power to help you get through the craving until it passes.

There is no such thing as a craving that doesn't wear itself out. Most people never realize that. They either give in to the craving as soon as it surfaces or fight it and end up exhausted. They can't see that cravings usually exit before long if they're denied attention. Another effective postponement technique is also significant in getting to Point Zero. That is learning to sit with your feelings.

SIT WITH YOUR FEELINGS

Long ago there lived a woman who believed that her house was possessed by demons. She called on the local priest to exorcise them. The priest performed the proper rites, but within a week the woman was again at the rectory gate. "My house is once more possessed!" she cried. The priest performed the ritual a second time and instructed his parishioner to return home.

Not a day had passed before the woman beseeched him a third time to cleanse her house. This request the good father refused. "The terrors that alarm you," he told her, "are less within the walls of your house than within those of your mind. You must confront these spirits yourself."

"But won't you give me something to help, a vial of holy water or a sacred crucifix?" the woman pleaded.

"I will give you something," the priest replied. "I will give you a holy stool." He took from the corner a simple wooden hassock. It didn't look particularly holy, but the woman took it nonetheless. When she entered her house, demons abounded from the cellar to the loft.

"I am lost," she thought. "Even with this holy stool as a weapon, I could never fight them all." She sat on the stool to await her fate, but the instant she was comfortably seated, the demons disappeared. The woman was convinced from that day forward that the cleric's gift indeed bore Divine Power. The priest, however, knew that her demons departed simply because she had been willing to sit with them. And he missed his favorite footstool for the rest of his life.

FOR ALL OUR CONTEMPORARY SOPHISTICATION, many of us are terrified by "demons." The ones we fear are not supernatural, they're our own feelings. We label some as negative—grief, remorse, anger, wounded pride—and feel justified in avoiding contact with them. Sometimes, however, we're equally uncomfortable with positive emotions. We're cautious about accepting compliments (we may not deserve them), feeling too good (we might jinx it), or even loving someone (they could go away). A tried-and-true way to keep from feeling anything is to overeat. You've heard the phrase, "to stuff your face." Well, it could as easily be stated, "to stuff your feelings."

The surest road for getting past anything difficult or emotional is the road that leads you through without turning to food. In other words, sit with your feelings. The feelings may have to do with a major life upheaval. Sit with them. More likely, the feelings you'd prefer to eat into oblivion result from everyday annoyances, nuisance situations, solvable problems that will work out whether you choose solution A or solution B. Whether you're meeting tragedy or trivia, you can sit with your feelings without food in your mouth. Each time you do this, the intensity of your desire to abuse food will mitigate and you will, perhaps without even knowing it, be inviting precious serenity into your world.

What it means to sit with your feelings is simply that: to be with them, to feel them, to come to know that they're not demonic forces but rather healers in their own right. Grief is a perfect example. Feeling grief, although certainly not enjoyable, is our part in the necessary process of recovering from a loss.

Episodes of grief are precisely timed as if the body and mind share a well-set clock. You cannot grieve too much at once. There is some grieving now, some later. Eventually, when the process has been allowed to complete itself, there is no further need for it.

Other emotions operate similarly. Anger fades. So does elation. They come to pass, not to stay. Every emotion has a purpose and a duration. To get in touch with these, understand them, act on them when appropriate, and then let them go, it is necessary to be present to them. You can't do that while eating a hero sandwich, opening your mail, and watching the evening news. You do it by releasing the need for doing altogether and allowing yourself to simply be.

In our society-wide hastiness, it's easy to misinterpret feelings. What felt like hunger may be anger, shame, or fear. These feelings can manifest as a cold, empty sensation in the pit of your stomach. It's no wonder they are confused with the need for food. Lots of feelings can similarly be lost in translation. What seems like anger toward one person, for instance, may turn out to be anger toward someone else or toward ourselves. What came to us as tension or anxiety could be the need to cry or talk or get a hug. In sitting with our feelings, we pay attention to them, the way a wise parent knows how to pay attention to an unruly child, to learn what's behind the behavior.

Ideally, giving this sort of attention to feelings means taking some time to sit quietly and purposefully with whatever is going on inside you. This is a skill that will take some practice. You begin by not eating for the time being and choosing to do something with less potential for avoiding your feelings. Talking with an understanding person can be a godsend, as can writing in a journal, taking a walk, working in your garden, or availing yourself of a massage or some other sort of calming bodywork. Eventually, you'll be able to sit, on a borrowed footstool maybe, with whatever is happening in and around you, and you won't be afraid. As you open yourself to what you feel, you'll find that you become open to what you need. It may be a counselor or a day off or more fresh fruits and vegetables in your diet. You'll become aware of these things. What's more, you'll see that you get what you need.

I can remember when the prospect of voluntarily feeling what I was feeling without deadening it with food seemed about as likely as paying off the national debt from my Christmas savings. With enough reassurance from people who had done it, though, and with bits of practice whenever I could get it, I came to welcome opportunities to be present to my own interior life. It isn't always easy, but when you know that the only dependable way out of uncomfortable feelings is moving through them, the process becomes far less difficult to embrace. Fears decrease and boredom disappears. Problems cease being crosses to bear and become bridges to cross. And you'll come to expect something wonderful on the other side.

MAKE PEACE WITH THE PAST
• •

A Zen story has it that two Buddhist monks were traveling on foot from their monastery to another in a neighboring town. To keep their vow of silence between sunrise and sunset, they walked wordlessly, reverently. After a few hours, they came to a flooded crossing. A finely dressed young woman was attempting to get to the other side, but there seemed no way for her to do this without soiling her garments from the water and mud. Seeing her plight, one of the monks wordlessly approached her and, lifting her carefully, carried her across the rivulet. He then continued his silent journey. When darkness fell, the second monk admonished him, "I am shocked that, given our vows of purity, you blatantly touched a woman today!"

"It is true," the first monk replied, "that I carried her in my arms over the water. But you, my brother, have carried her in your mind all day."

WE'VE ALREADY TALKED ABOUT LIVING IN THE PRESENT. We don't take the first bite of a binge today. We sit with our feelings in this situation. To place ourselves firmly in the present, however, requires that we be at peace with the past. We cannot move gracefully through a current experience while lugging burdens of judgment, disappointment, guilt, and resentment—which, if examined, would prove to be burdens of antiques. Like the accusing monk in the story, though, we can carry these burdens all day, and sometimes all our lives.

To deal sanely and compassionately with the past and with all the people in our lives, half of the anonymous programs' Twelve Steps are devoted to personal inventory and personal peacemaking. Reread steps 4 through 9 in The Twelve Steps on page 243. You'll see that they begin with a thorough stocktaking (making a searching and fearless moral inventory) and a sharing of what is discovered with oneself, another person, and a Higher Power.

It's important not to confuse this kind of inventory with something else, or to skip over it because you have done something similar before. Taking an inventory is not an excuse for putting yourself down or blaming yourself for every woe in the world. In fact, a tendency toward excessive self-blame may come out in an inventory as something you wish to be free of. The inventory is not a confession in the way you may know that term because you won't be looking for rules you have broken. Instead, you'll find the actions and inaction that you are uncomfortable with, that you wish you could change, and that have led or could lead you to unnecessary food.

The inventory is also not a digging for deeply buried psychological paraphernalia as you might discover with a professional in psychotherapy. Surely insights will present themselves that will be enlightening to you, but you needn't worry about uncovering information that is too much to handle. You will be taking a straightforward inventory of your character the way a shopkeeper inventories goods in a store. It is a necessary part of your experiment in giving your poor, weary willpower a rest and in using Love's power from here on. There are many ways to take personal inventory, but the clear and basic procedure suggested in the book *Alcoholics Anonymous* is time-tested for success. The recommendation there is for a three-part inventory covering resentment, fear, and sexuality.

The resentment list has three columns: one for the person or institution resented, a second for what he, she, or it did to cause the resentment, and a third for what that effects in you. As an example, you might write that you resent (first column) your sister because (second column) she says you ought to lose weight, which affects (third column) your self-esteem.

The resentment inventory is both healing and informative. In column two, when you are able to write about precisely what your resentments are, you're also recognizing feelings that you may have denied for a long time. This is certainly healthy, but in itself it's not enough. To be free of resentment, it is necessary to see what's going on inside you, thus the reason for having column three. *Alcoholics Anonymous* cites self-esteem, pride, sexual relations, and finances as those areas of our lives most likely to be the wounded parties when we're holding a resentment.

Fear underlies a great many of the difficulties in all these areas. As you notice what comes out over and over in the third column, you'll be getting to know yourself much better.

The second part of the inventory is a list of fears. What are you afraid of? A sample fear list might look something like this.

- Losing my job
- Getting cancer
- Being fat forever
- Being hungry
- Flying
- Getting old

Whatever your fear, write it down. Keep writing as long as things occur to you. Nothing is too petty. If it comes to mind, it's in your heart, so put it in your inventory.

Our fears are also telling. The sample list shows insecurities around issues of health, safety, and finances. Some people have deeply embedded fears, which can require special work at times in a therapeutic setting. But many fear patterns can be traded for a faith response as soon as we decide to do so. Looking at the fears straight on is the first action necessary for making that switch.

The final part of the inventory concerns sexuality. Look at your past and present relationships and write about them. *Alcoholics Anonymous* suggests that you answer the following questions.

- Where had we been selfish, dishonest, or inconsiderate?
- Whom had we hurt?
- Did we unjustifiably arouse jealousy, suspicion, or bitterness?
- Where were we at fault and what should we have done instead?
- We subjected each relation to this test—Was it selfish or not?

You may find it helpful to add to these such additional queries as:

- When have I allowed myself to be hurt?
- Have I settled for sex when I was looking for love?
- Do I accept myself as a sexual being?
- Is there balance in my sexuality—that is, can I both respect and enjoy it?

Your answers are to provide insights into who you are, not provoke guilt feelings. This is an inventory, not the Inquisition.

If you do all three parts and you still feel that there's something missing, write whatever else comes to mind. And get a complete picture by topping off your inventory with a list of the things you admire and appreciate about yourself. False modesty is no good here. There are many splendid things about you. Write at least 10, or better still, 50. (And yes, it's okay for you to write that being a good cook is one of them.)

Then share the whole thing with another person. If you're in a Twelve Step group, you can do this with someone who has done it already. Otherwise, choose someone whom you trust to listen without judgment and accept you just as you are. Revealing the nooks and crannies of your soul to someone else— ideally someone who has seen and revealed nooks and crannies of her own soul—brings a tremendous sense of peace. Some people feel that they're truly a part of life for the first time after sharing their true selves with another person, as well as with themselves and with the God of their understanding.

As we continue with the Twelve Steps' suggestions for cleaning up the past, step 6 discusses our readiness to be without the character defects found in our inventories. It's amazing that we may actually want to hang on to shortcomings that have caused us pain and lured us into the kitchen. The fact is, we do often cling to them, just as we've clung to abusing food. There was a time when we needed that food because we didn't have anything better. Now we do.

Similarly, we no longer need many of the defects of character that we had thought were necessary to make it in the world. When our lives are based on spiritual principles, we can prosper without dishonesty or manipulation because we are able to accept success as Love reaching out to us. We can meet our needs without interfering with others meeting their needs because we will realize that there is enough fulfillment to go around. And we can feel satisfied with the food we need to be healthy and full of energy without looking to extra or inferior food that promises satisfaction but only bogs us down.

When we ask that troublesome parts of our personalities be taken away, we find that most are not so much removed as redeemed. A pushy personality becomes an outgoing, assertive one. Hypersensitivity is turned to sensitivity to the plight of other people, other creatures, and perhaps a heightened appreciation for art or nature. Low self-esteem becomes humble self-appreciation.

That word *humble* can have a red flag attached, and since step 7 is worded "Humbly asked [God] to remove our shortcomings," this word deserves some attention. We confuse it with humiliation, which food addicts have so often suffered, instead of humility, of which most people, fat or thin, addicted or not, could handle a hearty helping. Humility implies being who we are, not something other than that. And since we are already quite magnificent in our very humanness, why would anyone want to be more? Perhaps it's because we've often believed ourselves to be much less.

I like the status of humility conferred on Wilbur the Pig in the children's book *Charlotte's Web* by E. B. White. In it, Wilbur is spared from slaughter because his buddy, a literate spider named Charlotte, writes about him, by seemingly miraculous means, in her web. First come the accolades: Wilbur is "some pig," then he is "terrific" and "radiant." Charlotte's last weaving for her porcine companion is that he is "humble." That may have been the highest tribute of all.

Steps 8 and 9 on the Twelve Step path discuss making peace with other people or with ourselves regarding them. By going back to the inventory, you will see names of people you have hurt or with whom you have had some discord. Without assigning the role of villain to you or to them, you will see that these are people with whom there is outstanding acrimony that keeps you from balancing your life, the way that checks too long outstanding can keep you from balancing your account. Step 8 involves listing those people and step 9 involves making amends to those you've harmed, if that's possible, except when doing so would injure them or others.

There are plenty of reasons for wanting to bypass this step. You could say:

• More people have harmed me than I have ever harmed.
• He deserved what he got for what he did. (She did, too.)

• That creep is out of my life and I like it that way.
• I don't want to dredge up old dirt.
• It's easier to hold the grudge.
• This has nothing to do with how I eat.

I understand all these objections and each may have validity with the exception of the last. As human beings, human relationships motivate us more than any other factor beyond survival itself. We can deny their importance, but they are important nonetheless. Relations with other people have a great deal to do with what, when, how, and why a person with a food problem eats.

Be clear on what making amends entails. It is not groveling before another person, seeking his or her forgiveness, or re-establishing a partnership or friendship that has run its course. It is instead to amend the current, unsatisfactory situation.

I think of person-to-person amends as something like amendments to the Constitution. The people who drafted the original document didn't look at it afterward and say, "Oh, we left out freedom of speech and freedom of the press. Too bad." No, they amended what they had done with the Bill of Rights. That is what we need to do in our dealings with other people. We can amend (change, add to) our attitude or behavior toward them to make the relationship better.

Sometimes the best relationship is no relationship. That's fine. Your willingness to make each one the best that it can be is the goal. In the cases in which making an amend could honestly hurt that person or someone else, you can amend the situation within yourself. That is, you can choose to genuinely forgive the other person for his or her part in the situation, and grant yourself the same courtesy. If this is a person you do not see anymore, it may not be appropriate to seek him out. Nevertheless, if you should run into him at some point, you would have already instigated a healing of the past.

In some cases, amends can mean a simple apology. In others it can mean paying a monetary debt or making good on a promise. It can also mean putting your own name on top of your list and becoming fast friends with yourself. As you treat each situation in turn, you will find those "outstanding checks" coming in, and you'll be able to go to a new bank with evening hours and free checking. In other words, your life will be richer so your food won't have to be. Your life will be simpler so your food can be, too.

EXPAND YOUR COMFORT ZONE

There once lived a widow who was always happy. She was at home in the parlors of the wealthy and titled who sought her counsel and in the hovels of beggars to whom she brought cheer as well as bread and firewood. She delighted in the laughter of children and the ramblings of the elderly, in autumn leaves and spring flowers, in praying and in dancing.

In her town there lived a sorcerer. He was not an evil man, but he was selfish and used to getting his own way. He asked the widow for her daughter's hand in marriage. Now, she remembered something of marital bliss, and not wanting her daughter to wed an old man, refused him. The sorcerer was angry and sought retribution.

First he brought fevered sickness upon the woman, but she still had the joy of her daughter's sweet voice and her many friends to nurse her back to health. Next the sorcerer condemned her to poverty. She and her daughter learned to forage for herbs and wild berries. On this frugal fare, the woman's face lost most of its lines and an annoying bit of rheumatism left her.

Further angered by the thwarting of his revenge, the sorcerer thought long on the perfect spell. "This one she shall not overcome!" he vowed. Under the final curse, the woman was to have no peace, whatever the circumstances. She felt unfit to converse with the rich but too well-bred to associate with the poor, so she was lonely. Rain was too cold for her and sun too hot, so she stayed indoors. Work seemed drudgery and play foolishness, so there was nothing to fill her hours. The woman was happy no longer.

She begged mercy of the sorcerer. "You have taken from me my most precious gift, the ability to be happy in any company and in any occupation. This was the greatest bequest I had to leave my daughter. Without it, I see no other way than to take her life and my own."

The sorcerer's heart was moved to pity. "Woman, I see that what I seek is not your daughter's hand but her mother's secret." He lifted the curse and learned from the woman how to find contentment in every circumstance. And if you go to that town today, some will tell you that there is more to the story, that indeed the woman and the sorcerer were joined in marriage and lived many happy years together.

THE WOMAN IN THIS LITTLE TALE had a wide comfort zone. She found acceptance from everyone because she offered it to everyone, and she found delight in myriad activities because she looked for it in all of them. My friend Rita is like that. She loves opera, but she listens to country music on car trips so she can feel like a trucker. She knows about a million subjects, is convinced that she has never met an uninteresting person, and treats the world as if it were an amusement park to which she has a season pass. Rita has taught me a lot about comfort zones.

We all have one, that place or set of circumstances in which we feel safe, comfortable, and unthreatened. We stray from its center in situations that are unfamiliar or with which we have negative past associations. In these cases we tend to feel out of place; we may be uncomfortable with not knowing what to do or what's expected of us. It's only natural to feel more at ease in a friendly, familiar environment with people we know well, than in a strange place with strangers. Nevertheless, when we're grounded in the Love-based life, when we start each day from Point Zero, we carry an expandable comfort zone with us.

When you bring these principles to life by living them, you will find that your serenity will no longer need to come from personal charm, although you may be charming, or from knowing the social graces, although you may be graced with every one of them, but from your Higher Power. You will be able to talk with your boss or a subordinate, the President or some freckled friend of your 10-year-old, and be genuinely interested in that person and genuinely secure in yourself. You'll be looking across at people instead of up or down at any of them.

The fine line between a frightening situation and an exciting one will blur, and your increasingly positive outlook will choose excitement over anxiety every time. Beyond this, however, you'll find that your need for excitement will decrease and your preference for serenity will grow. Because you'll become proficient at getting what you need, more and more serenity will become available to you.

Start where you are right now. Perhaps your comfort zone seems small. You may think that almost no place on Earth is truly safe unless you're armored with food or protective layers of fat. Don't despair if you feel that you're starting from the bottom. Start. Create your own safe, nurturing, binge-free, guilt-free comfort zone. At first, this may be a private spot just for you. Then you can gradually expand it to include one other person you trust, then others.

Your comfort zone may well be much broader than this at the outset, but some places or activities may still seem unsafe: supermarkets, interpersonal confrontations, speaking before groups. Allow your comfort zone to grow. If you need to buy groceries, talk with a co-worker about a potentially volatile topic, or give a 20-minute talk, use the same techniques you did for sitting with your feelings—only this time you're accepting outer situations in the same way that you accepted inner ones. In this case, instead of quietly being with your feelings, you can act in any given instance, with your feelings or even in spite of your feelings.

As you incorporate honesty, honest eating, facing feelings, and letting go of the past into the framework of your life, your comfort zone will expand automatically. You will find yourself in possession of a degree of poise that may surprise you. You might attribute it to a new haircut or to taking vitamins or losing 10 pounds, and if that helps, well, here's to haircuts. But as you encourage the flowering of your spiritual self, you will come to see that that is the key to your becoming more and more relaxed with whatever the day presents.

No one has nonstop equanimity, but yours can increase exponentially as you come to accept yourself more and more. As you do that, you will also come to accept what is going on around you for precisely what it is at the moment, even those things that need to be changed. The more you are able to accept the way things are, the larger your comfort zone will become. This in no way means tolerating abuse or settling for less than you need. On the contrary, it means finding a centered spot in the midst of any circumstance. From that zone of comfort, from Point Zero, you can enjoy the positive and deal wisely and rationally with any negative elements that present themselves.

When my precocious daughter was in kindergarten, I commented to her that a certain minor difficulty was really a blessing. "Was it a blessing in a disguise?" she wanted to know. There is a place where the disguised ones are as valuable as the others, and blessings of every sort abound. That place is Point Zero. You may be there now as you read this book. If not, know that you're on your way.

A MENTAL MAKEOVER

UNPRODUCTIVE, NEGATIVE THOUGHTS can be turned into powerful, positive ones.

Here are some examples of typical subzero self-talk and the respective Point Zero responses.

SUBZERO THINKING	POINT ZERO RESPONSES
I don't measure up.	I am adequate and more than adequate.
I don't belong here.	I am at home in my life and in my world.
Other people have their lives together.	I refuse to compare how my life feels to how their lives look.
There's some secret to happiness, but I don't have it.	Discover something to be happy about every day.
If I could lose weight (or stop purging), my life would be in order.	I live in an orderly way at my present weight.
If I didn't manage everyone and everything, there would be chaos.	I take care of my own life and leave the rest to God.
If you knew the real me, you wouldn't like me.	I am a likable person through and through.
Things have been too good; I'm due for something awful.	Things are good and I am grateful.
Whatever it is, it's my fault (or your fault).	My focus is on solving the problem, not assigning blame.
I'm afraid of what will happen.	I live in the safety of the present moment.
I don't know what to do.	I do the next thing indicated.
I can't keep up the facade.	I am who and what I am.

If you would change, I could.	I make the changes that are right for me regardless of anyone else's behavior.
I know what to do, but I'm doing just the opposite.	I know what to do and, alone or with help, I do it.
I can't (try, start, risk, succeed), so I won't.	I can (try, start, risk, succeed), and I'm doing it.
I'm tired and I haven't done anything.	I have plenty of energy to do what is mine to do.
If I'm not perfect, I'm a failure.	I am a perfect human being and perfect human beings have imperfections.
Nobody else is like me. I'm a special case.	I am a member of the human family. I'm a special person.

FOOD FOR POINT ZERO

- Eating everything on your plate will not help a single starving child. Throwing away food that you don't need is not terrible. If the food is good for your dog, feed it to the dog. If not, feed it to the Earth via a compost pile.
- It is possible to get a fix from not eating just as it is from eating. Do you get high from dieting or missing meals? Look at your behavior around food. The goal is balance, to get food into its proper place in your life as a whole. That will mean diminishing its importance overall and not looking to food, either more or less than you need, to feel better.
- You can prepare a meal without eating half of it in the process. At first you may wish to cook from recipes so you'll know the seasoning is right without tasting. If you do need to taste, do so at the end of the cooking process. A tiny taste will tell you all you need to know.
- If some food situations are particularly problematic, you can ask those around you for help. As an example, if you've gotten into the habit of fin-

ishing off your children's leftovers while you clear the table, make getting the dishes to the sink or dishwasher and the scraps to the compost heap or garbage disposal their job, not yours. Eventually, that kind of temptation may not matter, but as long as it does, give yourself a break.

- There is no magical food that will make you lose weight or that will take away your appetite forever or anything like that. Appreciate what is seemingly magical about food: that it can be transformed into what's needed to fuel one very important organism—you. If your relationship with food has been awful, approach it with an attitude that's more awe-filled.

- Food is neutral, like water. Water is a necessity, but it can also flood your basement, shrink your best pants, or even take your life. Similarly, food becomes a problem when it is misused or ill-chosen. For this reason, your focus needs to be first on your life, then on your food.

- Wanting to lose weight is not the same thing as wanting to stop eating for a fix. A heartfelt desire to live fix-free carries in itself tremendous spiritual power because it implies a willingness to live by the laws of nature and, if you will, of God. There's nothing wrong with desiring to lose weight simply to have a slimmer body, but spiritually, it's about on par with wishing for a trip to Las Vegas.

- You can say no to any food offered to you by any person on this planet. If that person is offended, there is a problem, but the problem isn't yours.

FOUR
Looking In, Reaching Out

SPENT YEARS OF MY LIFE LOOKING FOR A BALANCE. I WANTED the scale to balance on one number rather than another. But like watched pots that won't boil and counted chickens that refuse to hatch, that balance eluded me until another, more important balance was struck. That is the balance between my inner world and my outer one. In active food addiction, one of those invariably outweighs the other. Often I was caught up with work, other people, and frenzied activity, thereby avoiding who I really was. At other times, I stayed alone as much as possible, shielded with food, books, and television. The built-in isolation of eating for a fix kept me separated from both the richness of my interior world and of the world around me.

If you relate to that kind of separation, you can rest easy knowing that with every day you live fix-free, you will gently come more fully into the stream of life in a balanced way. Conversely, as you invite that fullness of life into your own experience, you will find that abstinence from unhealthful eating gradually becomes natural and effortless. The task at hand has two parts: first, to look within through self-study, meditation, and prayer, then to reach out to others in friendship and service.

Life is filled with such inner and outer dualities. Creativity, for example, needs an idea (internal) and expression (external). Each depends on the other. Artists don't lose their talents when they express them. On the contrary, every poem or painting refines, perfects, and intensifies the creative capacity of the person responsible for it. Along with your growing realization of your spiritual nature, your positive feelings and exuberance will actually increase as you share them with those around you and express them in all you do.

Understandably, a lot of people regard spirituality as optional at best because it appears to have to do only with intangibles. For addicts, however, those intangibles can get solid pretty fast. We require an active, sometimes intense, spiritual life in order to have a life worth living. Our spirituality provides us with the wherewithal to deal with food, people, and problems just as surely as our work provides us with money for paying bills and going shopping. Declining a spiritual life would do to our recovery what declining an income source would do to our buying power.

You may already acknowledge your spirituality. To bring it to bear on your food situation, you may need simply to expand that acknowledgment, to realize that food addiction affects the soul as well as the body and that it is important enough to take to your God. Or perhaps you don't buy all this spirituality stuff. Self-examination may seem unnecessary and prayer ridiculous. Why pray if there's no one to hear? Why share and risk rejection? I think that we look inside when we're tired of living with a stranger. We pray when we're tired of living alone, and we share because we're grateful that we're no longer tired.

You see, spirituality is like food and exercise. If you don't eat, you can survive on fat reserves but not indefinitely. If you don't exercise, your muscle tone will last for a while but not for long. Going within provides you with spiritual food; giving to others is your spiritual aerobics. They work together.

SPECIALIZING IN TRANSFORMATION

THIS IS STILL ANOTHER DIFFERENCE BETWEEN what we have done together so far and the other approaches that you've probably taken in an attempt to change the way you eat. Where diets and their kin focus on food, we've focused on you and your relationship with the spiritual power within you that specializes in transformation.

That goes far beyond the mere restructuring of your body. When a physical change happens without the involvement of the rest of your being, it's doomed from the outset. It's no wonder that 90 percent of the people who lose 25 pounds or more regain it within only two years. They don't realize that the body is, ultimately, a reflection—a reflection of what is going on inside: emotionally, intellectually, and spiritually. A physical body of the size you fancy hasn't a chance of staying that way without the support of your heart, mind, and soul, without the support of your entire way of life.

Weight loss by itself is like winning the lottery. It's terrific, but many lottery winners, like weight losers, wake up at some point where they started, wondering what happened. What happened is that the recently rich aren't always able to develop the attitudes (emotion), knowledge (intellect), and/or consciousness (spirit) necessary to maintain prosperity. And the suddenly svelte usually lack the attitudes, knowledge, and/or consciousness to maintain bodies of pleasing proportions. (Attitude and consciousness are far more important than knowledge. With the right attitude and consciousness, you'll get the knowledge you need. You can, however, be a literal information bank on diet, nutrition, and the like and still be caught in the morass of compulsive eating.)

Both lottery winners and the weight losers experience a change in form—net worth or gross poundage—but transformation is more than that. Dr. Wayne Dyer, who does a lot of work with this idea, defines transformation as going beyond form. That's what your Love-powered release of weight will be: a going beyond the form (this size or that, a larger waist measurement or a smaller one) to become the sort of person whose desires, preferences, and practices sustain a healthy, attractive body as a matter of course.

You have already realized that you can no more control your weight than you can control your grown children or the commodities market. What you are now doing instead is becoming someone for whom weight control is no longer an issue. This proceeds from the inside out. You've built a strong foundation while following the suggestions in the preceding chapters. Now you'll be looking at ways to guarantee daily renewal of the spiritual fitness necessary to keep food addiction at bay. That guarantee depends on keeping your life in ethical order, developing a viable relationship with the God of your understanding, and being of service to others as you put your entire life on a spiritual basis.

Remember that spiritual, as we're using the word, can be defined as transformational. It certainly can imply religious convictions, but for the purposes of leaving your addiction behind you, generic spirituality works just as well. Your personal spirituality can be nurtured on a continuing basis with the final three of the Twelve Steps. The first of these, step 10, states: "Continued to take personal inventory, and when we were wrong, promptly admitted it."

ROUTINE MAINTENANCE

THINK OF YOUR CHARACTER AS A CAR. The moral inventory of step 4 was a major tune-up: This ongoing, daily inventory is routine maintenance. When you take care of your car, you don't have to worry about driving it. When you take care of your life, you don't have to worry about living it.

Because we learn from mistakes, we're bound to make them as long as we're alive. We can't afford to deny them, rationalize them, or wallow in them. That's what ongoing inventory is about. The book *Alcoholics Anonymous* gives explicit instructions for how to go about this: "We continue to watch for selfishness, dishonesty, resentment, and fear. When these crop up, we ask God at once to remove them. We discuss them with someone immediately and make amends quickly if we have harmed anyone. Then we resolutely turn our thoughts to someone we can help."

This is gratis guilt prevention. A mistake is like an accidental spill. Guilt is the stain that develops if it isn't cleaned up. Making instant amends most profoundly benefits us, but it also does wonders for our relations with others. We don't allow minor slights and misunderstandings to escalate into major ones. We don't allow the time to elapse in which our difficulties with another person could be taken to gossip court and tried by a jury of our peers.

Many people find it helpful to take a nightly mini-inventory in addition to their daily lookout for selfishness, dishonesty, resentment, and fear. This inventory is a mental scan of the preceding waking hours to detect any unresolved disharmony or discomfort. Sometimes all you need to do here is forgive yourself and go to bed. Perhaps you'll want to offer a situation to your Higher Power or talk it over with someone. If something needs to be done about it tomorrow, make a note to that effect in your mind or in your journal, and tuck it away for the night.

QUALITY TIME WITH YOUR HIGHER POWER

B EFORE YOU GO TO SLEEP, spend a few quiet minutes with yourself and your Higher Power. Have another quiet time in the morning before the demands of the day take all your attention. This is when you indulge yourself in the peacefulness of prayer and meditation. Certainly you can "pray without ceasing" in your thoughts and actions overall and maintain the Buddhists' attitude of mindfulness, a meditative appreciation of every moment as you go through your day. But setting aside some minutes specifically devoted to your inner life is necessary, too. You have quality time with your children. This is quality time with your God.

The Twelve Steps discuss this in step 11, which says, "Sought through prayer and meditation to improve our conscious contact with God as we understood Him, praying only for knowledge of His will for us and the power to carry that out."

For many people, this is an impelling invitation just as it's written, but if the word *God* doesn't give you feelings of warmth and peace, use another name or another image. Change "His will" to "Her will" if that, as the Quakers would say, better "speaks to your condition."

A recovering alcoholic who writes anonymously as Rachel V. addresses this eloquently in her book *A Woman Like You*: "In [Alcoholics Anonymous] meetings now, I say that I'm promiscuous with God. I call on everyone: the Blessed Mother, the Lord Buddha, God the Father, Jesus Christ, Tara, the Holy Ghost, my grandmother, Inanna, Kuan Yin, Isis, Ishtar, Kali, Sophia, the Shekina, anybody and everybody. I need all the help I can get. I'm sure that God understands. My life is evidence."

Striking a balance between our inner and outer worlds can reveal that kind of evidence in any of our lives. Prayer and meditation symbolize the balance exquisitely, because in them we reach out to a Higher Power by looking within to the place in ourselves where that Power resides. There is a myth in Hinduism that tells of the upset experienced by the gods after they created humans. They were afraid that this cocky species would discover divine truth and that people would then become gods themselves. To avoid being overtaken by upstarts, the gods tried to figure out where they might hide the truth out of humans' reach. If they hid it in the treetops, a person could climb there. If they hid it at the bottom of the sea, someone would dive down to discover it. The cleverest of the gods finally suggested, "Let us hide the truth deep inside every individual. That is one place they'll never look."

Well, sometimes we do. That's what prayer and meditation are about. Basically, prayer is talking to God and meditation is letting God answer. There is no single right way to do either one. If you follow a religious teaching, there is likely to be a wealth of information about prayer and meditation within your own tradition. As you explore it with renewed appreciation, you're apt to see a depth and beauty there that may have eluded you before. If you don't have such a tradition to draw on, you can still rest easy knowing that prayer comes naturally to human beings as long as we don't get caught up in trivialities such as "thee" and "thou" and "ah-men" versus "a-men." If prayer is new to you, if you haven't tried it lately, or if you're feeling inhibited or skeptical about it, here are some suggestions.

How to Talk to Your Higher Power

Talk with your Higher Power the way you would talk with a trusted friend. Don't bother thee-ing and thou-ing. Just talk—silently is fine. Share what's going on with you. If you feel foolish doing it, talk about that, too. You can share anything—even if it seems petty or you think that God would disapprove. The loving God you're coming to know does not disapprove of you.

- Read or commit to memory a couple of prayers that appeal to you. Think about the words and what they mean.
- In the morning, offer your day to God. Ask for help with your eating and for the decisions you will make that day. Ask to remember in the midst of all your activities that you're no longer by yourself.
- Write to God. Put your thoughts, feelings, concerns, and delights down in a notebook or journal.
- Start a prayer list or a prayer box. Put the names of people who are on your mind or situations beyond your control on a list in your notebook or in a small box or jar. Think of these names or situations when you have some quiet time.

- Pray with your voice, your body, and your creativity. Song, dance, and art can be powerful prayers.
- Spend time in nature. Reverence is an effortless part of that.
- Pray with someone else. This can be extremely uncomfortable at first, but if you persist with it, you'll find a special relationship developing not only between you and your Higher Power, but between you and the person with whom you're praying.
- Explore affirmative prayer. Affirmative prayer is aligning our thoughts with God's through statements of divine truth. It's a way of opening ourselves to the blessings we've been ignoring, but which are immediately available to us. Affirmations are positive statements like, "God loves me, so I love and care for my body."

Most of us are used to praying for things, even bargaining for something like, "Get me out of this one, and I'll do volunteer work 22 hours a week for the rest of my life." We have treated God like a celestial Santa Claus, and when we don't get all the goodies on our list, we assume that prayer doesn't work or even that there is no God. It doesn't take much logic, however, to see that praying for things or for specific outcomes couldn't work in an orderly universe. I could pray for my side to win the war or the football game and you could pray for your side to win. Is God supposed to play favorites?

Or someone could pray to lose weight while eating a banana split and planning to have another. That's asking for a circumvention of natural law and is about as absurd as praying, "You know, God, I'm really sick of all this gravitational pull. How about letting me float around 50 to 60 feet above ground for a while?"

Besides, praying for things and automatically getting them would mean avoiding the lessons we're here to learn. Learning from life is as inviolable a principle as the laws governing gravity or the metabolizing of that banana split. This may well be why step 11 includes the phrase, "praying only for knowledge of His will for us and the power to carry that out." Now that can be horrifying. It's fine to let God have the cycles of nature and the orbiting of planets, but when it comes to my life, my relationships, and certainly the size of my jeans, I ought to know what's best! But you know what? I didn't know what was best all the time and I still don't.

Of course I can set goals, make choices, and steer my life in the direction that seems to be the proper one based on my intelligence, experience, and common sense. But intelligence, experience, and common sense aren't enough for a truly successful life. It also takes uncommon sense, intuition, and sometimes nothing short of Divine Providence. All prayers are answered, but sometimes when we pray for what we want, the answer is no. When we pray instead for the will of the God that loves us in spite of anything, the answer is always yes, always right, and always best in the long run.

When I was still doing periodic binge eating, someone told me to stop praying for anything, even to get over my food addiction. "I only pray to be of service," she said. "Then I get everything else." I didn't trust that until I began to see it work in my own life. First, I stopped praying to lose weight. I prayed instead to live in keeping with the laws of life. The prayer was answered as the foods I selected changed and exercise I actually enjoyed became a routine part of my life. Obesity cannot coexist with that lifestyle. I didn't have to pray to lose weight or work to lose weight. I prayed for God's will and, as my friend had also discovered, I got everything else.

Praying for God's will is not ignoring our problems and distresses. *The Twelve Steps and Twelve Traditions of Overeaters Anonymous* explains, "Clearly, if we are to develop a vital relationship with a Higher Power, we will need to bring into our prayers all the things that concern us. We pray about these things, not so we can get our way but so we can bring our will regarding them into alignment with God's will." Lasting peace of mind and the ability to live fix-free depend upon that alignment.

INNER LISTENING

BUT HOW DO WE COME TO KNOW WHAT God's will for us is? Well, we ask for it in prayer—then wait for an answer. This brings us to meditation, the state of mental stillness in which the still, small voice may be heard. Sometimes called contemplation or contemplative prayer, meditation is found in all religious traditions and is also recommended by psychologists and health care providers as a means of stress reduction. Simply stated, meditation is mental focusing. The object of that focus may be a word or syllable, an object such as a flower or candle flame, a phrase from a prayer or a scripture, or simply your own breath as you sit quietly observing your inhalations and exhalations— breathing in, breathing out, one breath at a time, no hurry, no worry, nothing to do but sit, watch, wait, breathe, and listen. An easy beginning meditation is to count your breaths. Count 1 on the inhalation, and use a word such as *love*, *peace*, or *shalom* to mark the exhalation. Count 1, peace, 2, peace, 3, peace, 4, peace, and so on until you reach 10. Then start again. (If you hit 17 before you realize you've passed 10, gently bring yourself back to 1. You're doing fine.)

When your mind wanders to what's on your desk at work, bring it back: 1, peace, 2, peace, 3, peace.... When your mind wanders to what to wear to the party this weekend, bring it back: 4, peace, 5, peace, 6, peace.... When your mind wanders to world affairs, your father's surgery, or your teenager's Standard Aptitude Test scores, bring it back an focus: 7, peace, 8, peace, 9, peace, 10, peace.... Then start again: Inhale 1, exhale *peace*; inhale 2, exhale *peace*....

Do it for at least 10 minutes in the morning (mornings and evenings are best). And 20 minutes in the morning and evening would be ideal, but even a little meditation beats none at all. Your relief from addictive eating or obsessive weight control will come with living in the love you're offered by love's very source. There is no substitute for connecting with that source voluntarily, regularly, and repeatedly. This may seem like a lot to do, but after you've made a place in your life for prayer and meditation, you'll wonder what you ever did without them. By reading about them and talking with people who already practice these spiritual disciplines, you'll devise your own routine for getting your much needed inner nourishment.

Your way will fit your schedule and your temperament. I'll share with you what I do just by way of example. First, let me stress that I am not a marathon meditator. There are times when I find it boring and would rather get on with the real highlights of life, like bringing in the newspaper and feeding the cats. I do not hear voices, see visions, levitate, or get any other noteworthy amusement from praying and meditating, nor would I want to. But I am more peaceful than I used to be—and less afraid. My life works pretty well, and right now I'm thinking about writing this page instead of thinking about something to eat. I believe that a great deal of the credit for this goes to the little bit of silence I take for myself virtually every day.

I start my day by recalling, even before I open my eyes, the realities that govern my life as a food addict: I cannot control food—that's the Higher Power's department; I renew my commitment to letting that Power deal with my life and my food for the upcoming 24 hours. Once I'm officially awake, I try to get to prayer and meditation right away. It doesn't always work out this way, but letting too many other things interfere can delete quiet time altogether.

Some people have a special chair or even a special room for meditation. I'm less formal. I usually sit up in bed Indian-style and start by writing in my journal. If there's something on my mind, it gets prayed out in pen and ink. If I'm feeling sorry for myself, I make a list of things I have to be grateful for. If the day ahead seems complicated, I write out my supposed obligations and see which of them really need to be done and which don't. In this way I clear my brain just as orators clear their throats. Then I read something centering. I usually select something from one or two daily devotional books, but anything brief and inspirational will do. Then I close my eyes, check to see that I'm sitting in some semblance of erectness (I want to be alert for this), and allow my mind to mull over the words I've just read. When my thoughts go off in other directions, I bring them back to those words, to their ideas. Sometimes I need more structure and do the breath-counting meditation instead. In either case I finish with a prayer to do God's will that day. All of this takes about 30 minutes. Sometimes I cut it short. My best days are when I don't.

SPAWNING MIRACLES

AT NIGHT I THANK MY HIGHER POWER for the day. Some days have been filled with surprises and successes for which I am grateful. Other times I do well to say thanks that my food was okay and that the day is over. I often read a little nighttime thought from a book I like, but I don't have a bona fide bedtime meditation. At least I don't yet, but life is so much richer thanks to the modicum of inward turning I do already, surely any addition would be all to the good. Still, none of us needs to become a contemplative cleric to benefit from prayer and meditation. Concentrated quiet time at some point during the day and remembering the spiritual foundation of our lives and our recoveries the rest of the time are sufficient for spawning miracles.

Saying grace at meals is also especially appropriate for recovering food addicts. We can be thankful not only for having food to eat but for not abusing the food we have. If saying grace hasn't been a custom in your family, you may feel awkward about it at first, even about bringing it up with the people in your household. If that's the case, I suggest that you start to share a minute of silence before each meal. The people present can hold hands if they like. That minute may be used for a short prayer of gratitude, to remind yourself that the meal is in God's hands and you are, too, so you can eat without fear and without trying to meet emotional needs from what's on your plate. Those 60 seconds can also be a calming, centering time. Eating in that state of body and mind will make the food much more satisfying and it can even assist digestion.

Children are comfortable with graces and don't have nearly the inhibitions about them that some adults do. My daughter has taught me some lovely ones. This one comes from schools that use the Waldorf system of education founded by Austrian Rudolf Steiner: "Earth who gives to us this food, Sun who makes it ripe and good, Dear Earth, Dear Sun, by you we live; our loving thanks to you we give." She adapted another from Robert Lewis Stevenson's *A Child's Garden of Verses*: "It is very nice to think the world is full of food and drink and little children saying grace in every sort of holy place." (I'm also fond of the impromptu grace that I overheard from a woman as she entered a buffet line: "Okay, God, You're on.")

It also makes sense to have an after-meal prayer. When we binged, meals never stopped. A prayer can give parameters we need. A Protestant friend of mine attended a Catholic mass and took note of the priest's closing words, "The mass has ended. Go in peace." She turned that into an after-eating prayer: "The meal has ended. I go in peace."

Indeed, to go in peace is how we can best leave a meal, a meditation, or any other activity. The peace that comes from giving our food problem to a Higher Power and from practicing prayer and meditation comes to life when we express it. Remember that balance of our inner and outer lives? This is it: turning what we receive from going within into sharing, caring, giving, and growing in our world, our work, and our relationships.

Step 12 addresses this: "Having had a spiritual awakening as the result of these steps, we tried to carry this message to [others] and to practice these principles in all our affairs." Only this step includes the verb "to try." The others are quite clearly to be done, but because carrying the message implies a response from someone else, it can only be tried. What the other person does with it is up to that person.

If you've taken advantage of the tremendous help that's available by contacting other recovering food addicts, you know that people who are putting these principles to work for themselves have turned theory into fact in a most impressive way. We need to be shown that spirituality isn't just Pollyanna pleasantness but that it can actually bring people from obsession, obesity, and despair to lives that are in order, bodies that are healthy and comfortable, and outlooks that are hopeful with good reason to be so. You can in turn offer this to others.

You don't need to wait until you're thin (that will eventually happen) or until you're perfect (that will never happen) to be of service to someone else. When I first began to look for a spiritual solution to binge eating, I was put in touch with a woman who proved to be very helpful. We had a wonderful long-distance conversation and just before our good-byes she said, "Now call someone and give them whatever you've gotten from this talk."

"But I can't do that," I protested. "I just binged last night."

"There's someone out there who binged this morning," she replied. "You have something they need."

I did what she told me. I called someone who I knew used food the way I did and let her know what I had learned. Of course, I had to tell her that I was no expert and had only binged the night before. What I see now, though, is that no recovering addict is ever an expert. Any of us could choose to go back to old ways of thought and action and would be abusing food again in no time. Addicts who stay in recovery live in blessed moments, in the now, in a state of grace that keeps anxiety at bay. Because our new lives do not come from us as ego entities, we can only share with others in the company of good old humility.

Once your body is the way you want it, it is possible that you may want to forget where you came from. Years ago when I was still trying to control my eating with gimmicks and willpower, I lost weight through a commercial diet program and then got a job there. Everything went fine at first. But then I stopped relating to the people who came there for help. One day I unloaded to a co-worker: "I am so sick of being around fat women!" It wasn't two weeks before I was back to binge eating and a huge, rapid weight gain. At the time I hadn't a clue that I couldn't deal with those "fat women" because I was one of them. I had not accepted my addiction, my vulnerability, or to a great extent, my humanity. Going back to overeating was inevitable.

You can avoid such pitfalls by remembering Love as your power source. In a support group, you'll have ample opportunities to share, but life itself offers such chances, too. People will ask how you lost weight, or they'll comment on how much happier or calmer you seem. When they do, tell them a little. If they're interested, they'll ask for more. The idea is to offer what you have without force-feeding anyone. It's possible for your enthusiasm to come across as fanatical zeal, leaving the impression that you've seen the light and are ready to outfit everybody else with the sunglasses they're sure to need shortly. It's important to tone that down. When you're established in recovery, you won't be out to make converts or reach a quota, but simply to be a resource about what made the difference for you.

One way to avoid being pushy is to speak with "I" messages instead of "you" messages. An "I" message is saying, "I found that I needed a spiritual solution for my food problem" rather than, "If you'd get some spirituality into your life, you could stop overeating, too." You've heard the old adage, "Your actions speak so loudly I can't hear the words you say." It's true. Our actions are chattering all the time, sometimes in shouts, sometimes in whispers, but they're always heard. When you have had a spiritual awakening, your life itself will carry the message—not just to other food addicts but to everyone you contact.

HUNGRY FOR HARMONY

PEOPLE ARE HUNGRY FOR GREATER HARMONY, PEACE, AND UNDERSTANDING in their lives. Without these, some overeat; some overdrink; some overworry. Others stay moderate in their habits but never achieve more than moderate happiness. For people like these, just being in the same room with you once you have achieved inner peace could change their day. Being your friend could change their destinies. That's because disease isn't the only thing that can be contagious. Ease can be contagious, too. In the same way that looking to others to be role models and confidantes is invaluable in your recovery, being those things to other people will give your recovery strength and longevity.

It is that strong, day-by-day recovery that makes it possible to practice these principles in all our affairs. These principles will be obvious in your total way of living (for more on these principles, see chapter 9). Right now, though, while we're thinking about reaching out to others, let's consider how to incorporate our new ideals into our personal relationships. It begins with the inventory steps and making amends. As your recovery progresses, you will find yourself attracted to healthier relationships just as you will be attracted to healthier foods.

As you continue with persistence and the willingness to let your Higher Power work in every area of your life, you'll find yourself living what at first seems to be a paradox. You will love people more, but you'll be less attached. You'll be able to let go emotionally, freeing the people you care about to be themselves—their best selves. You'll stop trying to control other people, similar to the way in which you'll have stopped trying to control your food and your weight. You will accept people precisely as they are because you accept yourself precisely as you are.

There are plenty of good books available on improving relationships, and you may find them helpful in learning techniques for better communication and for relating more confidently to others. Strictly by virtue of what is taking place within you as you overcome your addiction, however, you can expect your dealings with those around you to improve. If they don't, you'll be equipped to take positive action. Unhealthy relationships that you may have tolerated before your Love-empowerment began will be like the clothes you wore then: They'll require some alterations.

Be patient with those who are watching you change. Remember that another's transformation can be threatening. Those you love need to know that you're not abandoning them as you become more fully who you really are. On the other hand, never allow someone else's fear of your growth to impede it. Your primary obligation is to your own unfolding. When you are committed to that, your commitment to your family, friends, and colleagues will have the best possible foundation.

Looking within for guidance and reaching out to get and give more of the same will make you a better friend and a better partner—not just to other people in your life but to yourself. You will treat others with fairness and respect, and you will accept no less from them. You'll be learning to love in the truest sense of the word because you'll be learning from Love itself. This is part of how the process works, part of the way your thinking/feeling nature must work if you are to live addiction-free. If you came to this way of life only hoping to lose weight, this is one remarkable bonus.

A PRAYER PRIMER

I WAS ONCE TOLD THAT IT'S IMPORTANT TO HAVE PRAYERS, poems, and uplifting quotations filed away in my memory bank because there would be times I would be alone with only what was in my mind. If I had stored away words of beauty and inspiration, they would be there for me. I have found that to be true. Some of those that serve me well are included here. Feel free to choose from these (many of which will be familiar to you) or find your own. You never need to use prewritten prayers in order to talk with your Higher Power, but they do make good company.

THE SERENITY PRAYER
God, grant me the serenity to accept the things I cannot change,
The courage to change the things I can,
And the wisdom to know the difference.

THE PRAYER FOR PROTECTION
By James Dillet Freeman
First published by Unity School of Christianity
The light of God surrounds me.
The love of God enfolds me.
The power of God protects me.
The presence of God watches over me.
Wherever I am, God is.

The Lord's Prayer

Our Father who art in heaven, Hallowed be thy name. Thy kingdom come. Thy will be done in earth, as it is in heaven. Give us this day our daily bread. And forgive us our debts, as we forgive our debtors. And lead us not into temptation, but deliver us from evil: For thine is the kingdom, and the power, and the glory, for ever.

A Sikh Devotion

From the Asi Ki War

Wonderful Thy word, wonderful Thy knowledge; Wonderful Thy creatures, wonderful their species; Wonderful their forms, wonderful their colors; Wonderful the animals which wander naked; Wonderful Thy wind, wonderful Thy water; Wonderful Thy fire which sporteth wondrously; Wonderful the earth, wonderful the sources of production; Wonderful the pleasures to which mortals are attached; Wonderful is meeting, wonderful parting from Thee; Wonderful is hunger, wonderful repletion; Wonderful Thy praises, wonderful Thy eulogies; Wonderful the desert, wonderful the road; Wonderful Thy nearness, wonderful Thy remoteness; Wonderful to behold Thee present. Beholding these wonderful things I remain wondering.

A Hindu Prayer

Lead me from the unreal to the Real.
Lead me from darkness to Light.
Lead me from death to the knowledge of Immortality.
May the entire world be happy.

A Prayer of St. Francis

Lord, make me an instrument of your peace.
Where there is hatred, let me bring love.
Where there is injury, let me bring pardon.

Where there is discord, let me bring harmony.
Where there is error, let me bring truth.
Where there is doubt, let me bring faith.
Where there is despair, let me bring hope.
Where there is darkness, let me bring light.
Where there is sadness, let me bring joy.
Lord, grant that I may seek not so much
To be comforted as to comfort,
To be understood as to understand,
To be loved as to love.
For it is in seeking that we find.
It is in forgiving that we are forgiven.
It is in dying to the things of self
That we are born to Eternal Life.

AN ANTHROPOSOPHICAL PRAYER
By Rudolph Steiner

May the events that seek me come unto me.
May I receive them through the
Father's ground of peace on which we walk.
May the people who seek me come unto me.
May I receive them with an understanding heart through the
Christ's stream of love in which we live.
May the spirits that seek me come unto me.
May I receive them with a clean soul through the
Healing Spirit's light by which we see.

THE TWENTY-THIRD PSALM

The Lord is my shepherd; I shall not want.
He maketh me to lie down in green pastures; he leadeth me beside
the still waters.
He restoreth my soul; he leadeth me in the paths of righteousness for
his name's sake.

Yea, though I walk through the valley of the shadow of death,

I will fear no evil: for thou are with me; thy rod and thy staff they comfort me.

Thou preparest a table before me in the presence of mine enemies; thou annointest my head with oil; my cup runneth over.

Surely goodness and mercy shall follow me all the days of my life: and I will dwell in the house of the Lord forever.

THE PROPHET
By Kahlil Gibran,
from On Prayer

Our God, who art our winged self, it is thy will in us that willeth.

It is thy desire in us that desireth.

It is thy urge in us that would turn our nights, which are thine, into days which are thine also.

We cannot ask thee for aught,

for thou knowest our needs before they are born in us:

Thou art our need;

And in giving us more of thyself thou givest us all.

THE GREAT INVOCATION
By Alice Bailey

From the point of Love within the Heart of God

Let love stream forth into the

hearts of men.

May Christ return to Earth.

From the center where the Will of God is known

Let purpose guide the little wills of men—

The purpose which the Masters know and serve.

From the center which we call the race of men

Let the Plan of Love and Light work out

And may it seal the door where evil dwells.

Let Light and Love and Power restore the Plan on Earth.

NATIVE AMERICAN PRAYER

Now Talking God
With your feet I walk.
I walk with your limbs.
I carry forth your body.
For me your mind thinks;
Your voice speaks for me.
Beauty is before me
And beauty behind me;
Above and below me hovers the beautiful:
I am surrounded by it,
I am immersed in it.
In my youth I am aware of it.
And in old age I shall walk quietly
The beautiful trail.

• •

TO KEEP A JOURNAL

THERE ARE MANY WAYS TO PRAY AND MEDITATE. You can be in your house or in a church, on the beach or on the bus. You can pray and meditate in the lotus position or while sitting in a chair, kneeling, or walking. And you can communicate with yourself and your God with thoughts or words, or on a sheet of paper or in your journal, or on the blank pages provided at the back of this book.

A spiritual journal entails much more than keeping a diary or calendar, although it can incorporate those functions. The real purpose of a spiritual journal is to facilitate your inner growth. How it does this specifically depends upon you and what you want to achieve, but a journal can be used in any of the following ways.

1. Write in it in the morning to become grounded in the day at hand. There's something about writing today's date that implies a commitment to the nonrefundable span of time you'll have to spend during this day.

2. Record your food, either as a flexible plan for the day ahead or in the evening as a record of the gift of sane eating you received.

3. Describe your feelings when you're feeling a lot of anything, even if you can't label the feelings right away.

4. Write about decisions you have to make. List the pros and cons of your choices. This will help to clear your thinking process.

5. Write down what you need to do for the day. If there are 44 things to do in a 24-hour day, laugh. Then make cuts.

6. Write out affirmations. It's fine to speak statements of universal truth, but when you write them, especially if you do it several times a day for a month or so, they become your statements of personal truth.

7. Write letters to God (instant delivery, quicker than e-mail).

8. Write down ideas that you see or hear and want to internalize. Whether the thought comes from great literature or a bumper sticker, put it in your journal and assume that it will find its way into your life.

9. At night, empty your day into your journal. Make note of what you learned and what you're thankful for. If you do a personal inventory in the evening, this can go into your journal, too.

The mechanics of keeping a journal aren't really important. You can buy very attractive, clothbound books with blank pages and write in those, but if you have a practical nature like I do, you'll prefer a spiral notebook that stays flat and provides you with lines to write on. Be sure to write with a pen that feels good in your hand and glides easily across the paper: You can't "go with the flow" when your ballpoint is sticking. And don't fret about spelling or punctuation—your English teacher retired.

Sometimes people are wary of keeping journals because of the personal nature of what might be written there. Fortunately, most of us either have lives that are much less interesting than we think or handwriting so poor that the curious wouldn't bother to decipher it. Unless you have special circumstances, your journal is probably quite safe in a drawer in your desk or nightstand. If you write something you'd rather no one ever sees, tear out the page and destroy it. It's yours to do with as you like.

You can also choose to share the contents of your journal with another person. Sometimes our true thoughts and feelings come out much more lucidly when we're writing in a journal than when we're trying to speak extemporaneously. A dear person once said to me, "You'd better write it down. I've known you to put your foot in your mouth, but almost never in your typewriter."

You can save each journal you finish and go back to earlier ones as personalized reference books for your ongoing growth. On days when you doubt your progress, old journals can be solid evidence of how far you've come. They're also testimonials to everything you've come through with the help of your Higher Power. You will appreciate this resource when you are faced with difficulties that seem insurmountable. On the other hand, the truly loving life is the one you live today. In this respect, an outdated journal is so much kindling.

If you can use a record of the past to enrich the present, keep your completed journals. Otherwise, clear away the space they take in your drawer and in your psyche. This is a new day. Write the date on top of the page. Claim it. It's yours.

MORE REVOLUTIONARY CONCEPTS

THE REVOLUTIONARY CONCEPTS introduced in chapter 2 had to do with you as a person and your relationship with food. The following ideas are revolutionary as well, but they pertain to you as a friend and partner and to your relationships with the people in your life. Read them every day this month.

- Recovery will touch every aspect of your life. You cannot change the way you relate to God, yourself, and food without also changing for the better the way you relate to other people.
- If you have tried to control your food and your weight, you have probably tried to control people, too.
- You have one life: your own. No one else's life belongs to you, not even your spouse's or your children's.
- You may truly believe that you know what other people should do, but that doesn't mean that they'll do it or even that it's your job to tell them. Just share your own experience.
- With the exception of extreme circumstances like violence or abuse, no one makes you feel one way or another. You are the one who decides how you'll feel.

- Pleasing other people is fine as long as it pleases you, too. That doesn't mean that you should never be self-sacrificing: Just be sure that you want to do something for someone else before you do it so you don't end up resenting it.
- You can listen compassionately to another person without feeling that you have to fix that person's life or situation.
- There is no better way to make a positive connection with another person than by being exactly who you are. You are the best *you* on record, and your genuineness will be recognized by the genuine self of another person.
- The way to avoid having misunderstandings in relationships is to have no relationships. Having challenges in a relationship does not prove you a failure; it proves that you and the other person involved are human.
- Your opinions are as valid, your needs as important, and your life as precious as anyone else's. (This is true now, regardless of anything you have done, anything that has been done to you, how much you weigh, or what anyone says or thinks of you.)
- What other people think is not of your concern. As long as you're true to yourself, let others think what they like. (They will anyway.)
- Not every relationship is meant to last forever, and even those that last change.
- Having a relationship with food is much less difficult than having a relationship with a human being. The latter, however, is more rewarding and won't give you heartburn.
- Addictive people can have more than one addiction. An addictive relationship—one that is damaging but seemingly impossible to change or end—can impede your recovery. If you suspect that you need professional help or group support in this area, get it.

STRIKING THE BALANCE

KEEPING YOUR RECOVERY STRONG and viable will rest on two responsibilities: continued surrender of your eating problem to a Higher Power and maintaining the balance of a healthy spiritual life and a healthy life, spiritually lived. The following suggestions may help you come to this balance of "looking in, reaching out."

Make personal inventory an ongoing practice. Be on the lookout for self-ishness, dishonesty, resentment, and fear. When you see these, let your Higher Power take them; discuss them with another person, make apologies or take other action if indicated; and set your mind on helping others.

Review your day before you go to sleep. Is there something you want to talk about with God or another person or would like to handle differently next time? Is there some situation left from today that you want to take care of tomorrow? What progress have you seen in yourself today? What is there in your day that pleases you or that you can be proud of? Thank your Higher Power, and give yourself some credit, too. You're doing great.

Pray and meditate every day. Take some quiet time for yourself. Prayer and meditation are simply an expansion of that. Use your quiet time to read something soothing or inspiring, to write in your journal, to read or say any prayers that are meaningful to you, to talk with God, or to tend to the specific devotions that may be part of your religious faith. Use some of this time for silent meditation, using the breath-counting technique or another method to still your mind and be open to your Higher Power.

Share what you have found with others. Sharing is offering, not forcing. As you recover, you'll find ways to share nonintrusively and beneficially, particularly if you're part of a support group. Remember, too, that your life itself carries the message to other food addicts and everyone around you.

Remember your new way of life in all your activities and relationships. As someone relying on spiritual truths to recover from food obsession, you will be living a spiritual life. This doesn't imply prudish piety. It does imply putting all your actions and your dealings with people on a spiritual basis. As you live this new way and make contact with your Higher Power in prayer and meditation, much of this will come to you intuitively. You will look for something of God in everyone around you. You will allow other people to be who they are. You will be able to accept others as they are and, perhaps especially, yourself as you are.

FIVE
The Gift of Choice

Y OU HAVE EMBARKED UPON AN INNER JOURNEY. Its destination—spiritual awakening—is not like a port or a station. You won't arrive, unpack your bags, and be done with it. It is instead the opening of a door to a new way of life, one lived on a daily basis, renewable every morning. And every morning a spiritual gift will be waiting for you, just as surely as if it were a wrapped package with your name on the tag. That is the gift of choice.

There is no choice in eating for a fix. We did it when we thought that we wanted to and when we knew that we didn't, yet the idea of refraining from it was paralyzing because we thought that it meant our choice would be taken away. In truth, however, it is only when we're set free from having to overeat or undereat, reward ourselves with food or punish ourselves with deprivation, that we really have a choice at all. Only then can we make choices about our lives—to treat ourselves well, for example—and about our food.

As a recovering food addict, you will need to learn how to use the gift of choice the same way you have learned to use tangible gifts, from your first bike to your personal computer. In the throes of the addiction, many choices were limited. You wore an outfit because it was the one that fit. Perhaps you took a certain job because you didn't feel good enough about yourself to apply for the other one, the one you really wanted. And if you're like me, you certainly ate one particular food or another not because you really wanted it or even because it tasted all that great, but because it was around or it was the one that offered the kick or sedation needed at the time.

In recovery, choices abound. With a reprieve from food obsession and a commitment to Love-powered rather than ego-powered living, you will be able to:

- Believe that you're okay because "God doesn't make junk"
- Experience compassion
- Express your feelings
- Accept life instead of fighting it
- Have fun
- Welcome supportive friends
- Go with love instead of fear into your world
- Feel good physically and emotionally
- Give to life and enjoy the rewards of giving
- Forgive yourself and others
- Ease up on yourself
- Reach out to people
- Take risks
- Find humor in almost every situation
- Look on the bright side
- Rejoice in others' good fortunes as well as your own
- Take good care of yourself
- Be grateful
- Delight in the little things
- Feel attractive
- Be honest
- Smile
- Look forward to every day
- Unleash your creativity
- Grow
- Learn from difficulties
- See the beauty around you
- Put more beauty around you

- Love
- Be happy

Can you see that all these are choices? Does it make sense to you that we can choose, for example, to be happy, or does it seem that happiness has to happen to us, that it is the result of a hefty raise, a smart purchase, or a fresh compliment? Of course these things give us a boost. It's wonderful when they happen. That boost, however, is not happiness. Happiness is far less flighty. It comes from within and depends on little else. It is a choice. This does not mean that there will never be challenges, dilemmas, problems, and losses, even major ones. Feeling frustration, anger, and grief regarding these is natural, but your underlying sense of well-being—real happiness—will still be with you if you choose to have it.

There certainly may be times when you'll choose to feel unhappy. That's all right. You may want to give yourself an unhappiness allotment of an hour or two, and then get on with whatever it takes to put you back in touch with the reality that you can indeed choose to be happy. "Whatever it takes" will probably be one of the same methods you're already using to postpone inappropriate eating: talking with another person, getting a change of scenery, or having a quiet time for prayer, journal writing, or meditation. Do what you need to.

It isn't always easy to remember that you're choosing your own feelings, but you can go on the premise that all these choices are yours. And you'll see that the premise is correct. The ability to make choices is a gift from Love to you, a gift for you to accept and direct at will. There are two choices, though, that recovering food addicts need to make each day. The first is to choose to remember that our lives have been turned over to the care of a Higher Power. If you're working through the Twelve Steps, you made your original decision to let that Power take care of your will and your life back at step 3. That step could be likened to deciding to take a job. Choosing each day to remember the decision to keep things in God's hands is like showing up for work at 9:00 prepared to do the best you can.

When you operate from the proposition that your Higher Power (be it God, Love, or your highest spirituality) is handling the outcome of situations, you can do what you do best: Take care of what is in front of you. Don't believe for a minute that this means resigning yourself to dullness, drudgery, and an uneventful life. When you team up with the power of Love, what will be in front of you to do will oftentimes surpass your wildest dreams. Of course, there will be some dullness, drudgery, and uneventfulness. A full life comes in all colors, including a little gray.

The second important daily choice for continued recovery is to choose to refrain from eating for a fix. You actively implement this choice every time you use the postponement techniques and every time you elect to sit with your feelings without something to eat, drink, or chew for the time being. Therefore, you are already aware that choosing to refrain from eating for a fix bears little resemblance to going on a willpower diet. Diets can, in fact, impede progress because they give the illusion that we can control our eating, which, for any true food addict, is a dangerous fallacy. What is required in terms of food choices is a new way of eating that arises from this new way of thinking provided by a spiritual approach to life.

As your recovery proceeds and you reconfirm each day your commitment to your Higher Power, you will experience with growing frequency that choosing not to eat for a fix won't even seem like making a choice. It will be a non-issue, in the same category as having to choose whether to buy a jet this month or a small island in the Caribbean. That degree of freedom is incredible for those of us who've had difficulty getting through just one hour without obsessing over food. Nevertheless, eating for a fix can be virtually guaranteed to any food addict who goes back to former patterns of thought and action. Therefore, whenever you keep harmful or unnecessary food out of your mouth—even if this requires no conscious effort because you simply don't want the food—you have already made the choice to refrain from eating for a fix. You are unconsciously acting on that, and your appetite itself has, in fact, responded to the choice you have made.

I call these times state-of-grace days because we don't have to earn them. We only have to accept them. Expect to enjoy ever greater numbers of these as time goes by. On some days, though—and in the beginning it may be all days— you'll still want to eat the way you always have. This is not terrible and it does not mean that you are a failure. It most likely means one of two things.

The first possibility is that there is something missing in your spiritual life. Use the opportunity to look at your recovery practices. Do you recognize that your own power is useless when it comes to food? Are you looking to your Higher Power for help? Are you willing to postpone the fix and sit with your feelings? Do you need to let go of some shame or guilt or resentment that hasn't been dealt with? Would it help to talk things over with someone? Do you owe amends? Have you been taking time for prayer and meditation? Are you sharing with others? Are you using spiritual principles in all aspects of your life, those that have to do with your eating and those that don't? Sometimes taking a single action to deepen your spiritual life can rid you of the most stubborn food craving. If you can't pinpoint exactly what's amiss, just do something. Take a half-hour for journal writing and meditating, or call someone you know who is having a difficult time and offer that person a patient ear.

A second reason why you may be experiencing the desire to overeat could be physical. Perhaps you recently ate a particular food that, for you, incited an obsessive pattern, or there may be a lack of balance in your physical/emotional self. The anonymous programs use the acronym HALT to remind their members not to get too hungry, too angry, too lonely, or too tired. When you want to extend a meal beyond reasonable parameters or eat what you know is extra, unnecessary food between meals, examine your life in terms of HALT. You may have two or three of the danger signals operating without realizing it. Take care of them. This is another reason to stay away from diets. On most of them, you're hungry from lack of food, angry about being on a diet, lonely because so much socializing takes place around food, and tired from lack of nutrients or from trying to restrain yourself.

On those hungry days, you'll need to make the conscious choice to refrain from eating for a fix—and you may need to do it more than once. The difference between choosing to abstain from damaging eating and using willpower to stick to a diet is surrender versus combat. When you surrender the inclination, desire, or compulsion to misuse food to the power of Love, the struggle is over.

A WILLOW'S FLEXIBILITY

YOU CAN SURRENDER PERFECTIONISM at the same time you surrender your compulsions to misuse food. When you are no longer eating for a fix, you will still sometimes eat more than you need. You might make a food choice

that you wish afterward had been different. When these things happen, you will
not have "broken your diet," because there is nothing to break. You will have a
willow's flexibility to withstand storms that would demolish an oak. Without
having to reach some nebulous state of perfection, either in your life or at your
meals, you will be living out your choice to be free of the food fix one day after
another.

Another choice that will be yours in recovery is that of choosing what you
will eat. You don't simply stop and stay stopped as you might with another addiction. You need to stop abusing food but still decide what to prepare or what
to order for breakfast, lunch, and dinner. Knowing what to eat and how much
can be scary. After all, food seems to have been the cause of so much misery.
How do you know that you can trust it or that you can trust yourself to make
decisions about it?

You may remember the times when you fasted or went on liquid diets,
only to find your peacefulness again broken when you had to return to eating
solid foods. Part of the appeal of such programs is that with them you don't
need to have anything to do with food—out of sight, out of mind, so to speak.
But just as you can't learn to swim on dry land, you can't learn to eat in a loving
way, or even come to know that it's possible, until you try it.

THE FREEDOM TO CHOOSE

THE INNER CHANGE YOU'RE OFFERED will render you capable of dealing
with life as it is. Part of this life—for human beings and every other animal on
the planet—is to eat. Although every addict who expects to get well must respect the severity of addiction, fear doesn't heal anybody. Love does the healing,
and Love and fear cannot work in the same space. If you are afraid of food, put
that on the fear list in your personal inventory and ask your Higher Power to
take the fear away. As St. John once said, "Perfect love casts out fear," and this
still applies. You can expect to develop a new, respectful but fearless attitude toward food.

If you started turning to food when you were a child, you evidently needed
it to shield you from things you feared or didn't understand. Some people with

eating disorders were physically, mentally, or sexually abused as children, but even in happy homes, some needs go unmet. Then, the food was a friend, a helper, a protector. It can't help you anymore and you don't need its brand of protection, but it can become a friend in a sane, mature way—the way you may now admire and enjoy a sibling that you envied or resented as a child. Your attitude has changed. Your attitude toward food can change as well.

As your attitude changes, you will make food choices from a different vantage point. When, for example, you were eating for emotional solace, you may have gravitated toward sweet, creamy foods that were usually high in fat and nutritionally marginal. With a different motivation for eating—the desire to nourish yourself for the healthiest, happiest life possible—you are a ripe candidate for an attitude adjustment. You will, in effect, be making a shift: Food will no longer get star status, either as a hero or a villain. It will instead play an important but low-key, supporting role.

You are in the ideal place for allowing your attitudes toward food to change because you have been working from the inside out, looking at yourself first, then at your food. Dr. Dean Ornish, author of *Eat More, Weigh Less,* uses an approach with his heart patients, many of whom come to him overweight as well, that includes the spiritual disciplines of yoga and meditation, group support, aerobic exercise, and a low-fat vegetarian diet. He explains the role of inner change in this way: "It's not enough to simply change behaviors without dealing with deeper issues. Telling someone who's lonely and depressed and isolated that by changing her diet, she'll live longer isn't very motivating. Who wants to live longer if they feel bad? So we address the emotional and spiritual dimensions of health and illness, not just the physical. When you feel happier and more peaceful, you tend to choose behaviors that are life-enhancing, rather than self-destructive."

There are many kinds of life-enhancing behaviors (see page 84). Right now, though, let's focus on choosing life-enhancing foods. Think about this concept for a minute. Life-enhancing foods should look good, smell good, and be appealing in their own right. Just because some food is low-calorie, low-fat, or supposedly good for you doesn't necessarily qualify it as life-enhancing. Do you have any childhood memories of having to eat liver or cooked spinach or something else you detested? You may have swallowed it and ingested some useful nutrients in the process, but it's doubtful that you felt your life had been enhanced.

My friend Suzanne is an inspiration when it comes to life-enhancing food. After she changed her attitudes through spiritual principles, she set about changing her food attitudes most decisively. She cleaned out her kitchen and got rid of everything that didn't add to the health of her body or the beauty of her cupboards. Most of the packaged snack foods went, along with the white sugar and bleached flour. She filled her shelves with tawny grains and colorful beans stored in handsome apothecary jars she had discovered at a yard sale. Fresh fruit was always ripening on her table or counter, and after she befriended an organic gardener, she learned to grow sprouts and dry apples and to notice sunrises, sunsets, and the phases of the moon. She started making juices from concord grapes and Rome Beauty apples and concocting colorful smoothies (blended fruit shakes) for breakfast. My friend who had already been beautiful to those who knew her became strikingly so to everyone she met. Her eyes seemed bluer than they had been before. Her skin seemed translucent. Her body responded to this treatment with glowing health and increased energy.

We influence each other more than we know. Whenever I'm tempted to throw something together instead of lovingly preparing fresh food, I think of Suzanne. Then the need to rush doesn't seem as pressing. I put away the can opener and get out the paring knife.

There is no single, rigid way to eat that is right for everyone. We have different activity levels and different ethnic backgrounds. We live in different climates and in different social environments. Nevertheless, physiologically we are quite similar. Based on that similarity, there are guidelines about eating that apply to humans as a species. It makes sense, for instance, to eat primarily the foods that come to us from nature rather than expecting the body to deal with synthetic substances it doesn't understand.

It is known, too, that a diet high in animal fats is the foremost contributor to heart disease, the number one killer in this country. It has also been linked with several kinds of cancer, diabetes, osteoporosis, and many other plagues of civilization, overweight included. People who choose natural foods that are low in fat are healthier, as a rule, than those who eat processed and high-fat foods. Their bodies are leaner, although they eat heartily. In parts of the world where this style of eating is the norm, obesity is virtually unknown. Recovering food addicts who eat in this way do not have to be concerned about their weight, about portion sizes, or about cutting back after weekends or holidays.

Combining a spiritual turnaround and this gentle way of eating brings this loving approach full circle. Spirituality is the inner side; gentle, natural food choices the outer. Those who make natural food choices find that these choices support and complement their total way of living.

It may well be that a new way of life deserves—and perhaps demands—a new way of eating. Explore your options. Experiment. Read the books listed on page 239. Use your head. Consult your heart. Talk with your doctor, with your friends, with your God. Your spiritual awakening will provide you with the gift of choice. Unwrap it.

• •

THE NOW CHOICE

W E CAN ACCEPT THE GIFT OF CHOICE only in the present moment. Certainly our lives are enriched by happy memories and fond hopes. We can learn from the past and we must plan for the future, but we're asking for trouble when we try to live in either one. Focusing on the past invites regret and remorse. Denying the present for the future asks for worry and anxiety. Why? Because neither the past nor the future is real. The only reality is this moment. Some people call this the eternal now.

We are thoroughly in the present when we are engrossed in a project and lose track of time. That's when we aren't judging ourselves, when we're not late or early, too young or too old; when we're not concerned about what we've eaten or how much we weigh or anything else. We are in the process of being alive. In even a long life, the hours of being fully, blissfully alive can be few indeed. For many people, most in-the-now time is enjoyed during childhood. Children are grounded in the present to a degree that can be unnerving to adults.

In recovery, we can reclaim a degree of this childlikeness in allowing ourselves to be thoroughly in the present. This concept is particularly important for people who have had problems with food. Food addiction is often accompanied by an ongoing neglect of the present, replacing the attention that today deserves with focusing on last year's thinness or next week's diet. I'm partial to the line in the Lord's Prayer that says, "Give us this day our daily bread." This day. That's it. For years I was unwilling to gratefully accept my daily bread: I wanted several days' bread with honey and butter and cheese.

Living in the now is one way to come to know through and through that this day's bread—and time and inspiration and whatever else I need—is here for me today. For today, I'm taken care of. So are you.

Growth in recovery is a daily proposition. We can no more live on yesterday's spirituality than on yesterday's oxygen. We claim today's spirituality by making the now choice, by choosing to remember that:

- This is the only moment there is.
- This is the only moment we have access to our Higher Power.
- This is the only moment we can refrain from eating for a fix—and this is the only moment we need to.

ACTIONS THAT WILL HELP CHANGE OUR ATTITUDES TOWARD FOOD

1. Allow an inner transformation to take place through bringing your spiritual life to bear on your life as a whole—eating included. Using the Twelve Steps is one proven way to do this.

2. Find at least one person, preferably a group of people, with whom you can talk about your attitudes toward food whenever you need to. As soon as you are able, provide the same sort of support for others.

3. Bring your Higher Power into food situations with you. You are not alone when you remember that the God of your understanding is with you all the time. This help is not only available in dramatic situations but at banquets, buffets, and when you're passing a bakery window.

4. Be grateful for your food. Say a prayer of thanks at meals. Remember the contribution of everyone and everything, from the earthworms to the farmers, from the retailer to the cook (even if that's you).

5. Select and prepare your foods lovingly. Think about what it means to serve food to yourself and others. You are providing physical sustenance that will become a part of your living body and the bodies of people you care about. You deserve the best and so do they. This is a sacred trust.

6. Choose beautiful foods and present them beautifully. Your tongue may prefer fudge to strawberries, but your eyes are partial to strawberries. Indulge them for a change. Experience your meals with all your senses. Eat slowly. Put flowers on the table and play soft music—not just for company, but for you.

7. Discover the clean delight of simple food. I remember the first time I had a cup of tea without lemon or cream or sweetener. I was amazed at how delicately flavorful it was, how interesting to taste something I had drunk many times before without really experiencing it. You can discover something similar with an unbuttered potato, a plain bowl of oatmeal, or air-popped popcorn. Food certainly doesn't have to be bland or dull, but it is curious that for people who supposedly love food, we don't actually know what most of it tastes like.

8. Learn to feel safe between meals. Sit with the feeling of not being full, the way you have learned to sit with other feelings. Don't get Spartan about it (that's the dieter's mentality or even that of people with anorexia), but get to know how it feels to not be digesting food all the time. Realize that you can be content without being full.

9. Conversely, experience fullness. It's easy to ignore the body's signals that say "enough." Some people think that the bodies of chronic overeaters don't even produce these signals anymore, but I believe that they're simply ignored. Listen for them. How does it feel to be full? You know, you're okay after a meal and you're okay before one. It's all right to have a full stomach or an empty one. All humans and nonhuman animals at times have one, at times the other. Join the biosphere!

10. Explore the world around you. Thinking about eating and thinking about not eating have taken up enough valuable time. It's a wonderland out there. What do you really want to do? Would you like to take acting lessons, learn to knit, play golf, work for a cause, speak Italian, write short stories? Do it—not after you've had something to eat and not after you lose 10 pounds. Do it now.

BEFORE YOU CHOOSE YOUR FOODS

B EFORE YOU CHOOSE YOUR FOODS, make this choice: Choose to love yourself with food. Many food addicts say, "When I was growing up, food meant love in my house," and they use that to rationalize overeating today. There's a hole in the reasoning, though. Maybe love was expressed to you as a child through food, but if you're abusing food now, you're abusing yourself. That's not Love.

Decide to love yourself with how you eat just as you're learning to love yourself with how you live. Some of the following suggestions will seem familiar. You may have even tried them. What's different this time, though, is that you are now engaged in a transformational process that is spiritual and thereby total. That transformation will make it possible for you to implement these suggestions, even if you have tried them and failed in the past. In fact, as your inner transformation continues, you'll see that you will be taking many of these measures without giving them any thought. You will read this list and say, "Yes, I'm doing that."

Eat without guilt. Guilt enjoys its own company. The guiltier you feel, the more you're likely to continue the guilt-producing behavior.

Eat for your health. Don't pass this one by because it seems so obvious. How many people do you know who truly choose their foods to bring about high-level health? Precious few. Be one of them.

Eat slowly. Even if you have only a half-hour lunch break, don't inhale your food. Chew it. Taste it. If meals are routinely rushed or interrupted (if you work on call or if you're the parent of small children), make a point of slowing down for the meals at which you do have that luxury.

Eat when you're calm and centered. If you're upset, don't eat, even if it's mealtime. Pray. Take a walk or a bath. Phone someone. Sane eating and inner turmoil are rarely found at the same table.

Eat the way that's best for you, regardless of others' opinions. The majority of people are far superior to the food they eat. Every human being is a divine creation entitled to the very best, yet most people in our culture eat quantities of fast, fragmented, and "foodless" food. When you stop joining them in this, they're liable to rib you about being a health nut or being on some foolish diet. You're neither; continue to do what's right for you.

Eat food prepared with love, care, and attention. When you are the chef, prepare your food in this way. When you eat out, choose places where you are most likely to get food that has had love, care, and attention given it. This doesn't have to mean always going to expensive restaurants. Many places are as concerned with these intangibles as with the special of the day: Look for restaurants that prepare their food fresh, that are privately owned and have the owners on the premises, and that specialize in natural foods. Many ethnic restaurants, particularly family businesses, are good places to dine.

Allow your tastes and preferences to change for the better. When you are committed to treating yourself well with the foods you eat, you are willing to make some changes, to try some new things. You probably won't like all of them and you don't need to, but you can allow your tastes and preferences to change, to appreciate new textures, subtle flavors, and lighter versions of dishes that otherwise couldn't offer you the love you deserve.

Let your food choices express who you are. You are a beautiful, healthy, compassionate, intelligent human being. Select foods that are beautiful to look at, smell, and taste; that contribute to your health; that express compassion to others; and that are the result of intelligent discernment.

These suggestions can more easily become a part of your thinking and thereby a part of your life if you turn them into affirmations.

1. I eat in love, not in guilt.
2. I eat for high-level health.

3. I eat slowly. There is plenty of time.

4. I eat only when I am calm and centered. (Or, I give myself the gift of becoming centered before every meal.)

5. I eat in the way that is best for me, regardless of anyone else's opinion.

6. I eat only food prepared with love, care, and attention. (Or, when cooking, I prepare food with love, care, and attention.)

7. I allow my tastes and preferences to change for the better.

8. I let my food choices express who I am. (Or, I make food choices that express beauty, healthfulness, intelligence, and compassion.)

SIX
The Love-Powered Diet

MOST PEOPLE WHO HAVE BATTLED FOOD have done exactly that: battled. But with the principles you have been incorporating into your thinking and living, the kitchen no longer needs to be a war zone. We've discussed the spiritual and emotional aspects of this new way of life first so that your food choices can now reflect those spiritual and emotional changes.

We're about to explore a lifesaving and life-affirming way of eating that I believe mirrors spiritual growth and emotional stability. It's a way of eating that also does your body good while sending feelings of deprivation packing. No style of diet, however, can cure a food addict. That's like saying that a drug can cure a drug addict. It will take more than an eating plan to heal the emotional wounds that you may have tried to salve with food. It is critical that you learn to live in conscious contact with the Love that is able to give you the emotional strength that no diet can provide. Love and learning how to reshape yourself from the inside out are your foundation.

This chapter is about the power of Love in making simple food choices. It is important to realize that when that power of Love touches you anywhere, it touches you everywhere. In this case, wanting to have it all isn't greed; it's good sense.

Before I begin to make my case for the way of eating that I have found to express Love in my life, let me be absolutely clear that you must choose a way of eating that expresses Love in your life. It is my hope that you'll read this chapter carefully and consider the points that it makes both philosophically and with regard to commonsense nutrition. Nevertheless, you certainly don't need another food plan imposed on you from some outsider. If you have had a long-standing food problem, you've probably studied as much about diet and nutrition as some professionals in the field. You can make your own healthy decisions in this area. You'll probably agree with many of the points you're about to read but may choose a different approach on others. This is all part of the gift of choice.

Now, what on Earth could Love have to do with what you eat? Chances are, it hasn't had much to do with it, and that is what put you in the pickle that led you to this book. Surely no loving God and no loving part of yourself wants you to be tormented by food cravings, subjected to depressing and even dangerous diets, or risking your life with morbid obesity or a binge/purge merry-go-round that ceases to be merry long before the ride is over. It also stands to reason that a loving God or your most loving self would be interested in your overall welfare and in the welfare of all people, all forms of life, and an Earth so nurturing to us that many call her Mother.

Because Love encompasses everything, nothing is unimportant, including tonight's dinner menu. Think about it for a minute: If you were pure Love, the loving parent of all life, how would you want people to eat? I wish that I could hear your answer. Perhaps you would want people to nourish themselves in a way that:

- Is generous, delicious, and aesthetically pleasing
- Promotes high-level health as well as normal weight
- Is economical and provides plenty for everybody
- Respects all life
- Is environmentally sustainable

That is the definition of the Love-powered diet.

Diet can be an ugly word, and sentences like, "I'm a fat slob and ought to go on a diet" or, "I was bad and blew my diet" are no less than obscene. I'm using the word quite differently here. The Love-powered diet applies to a natural, gentle style of eating that uses the "D" word in its general and nonthreatening sense, as when you say, "I make sure that my children get a well-balanced diet." What people eat is their diet. Depriving oneself in order to lose weight is dieting. What we're talking about is a way of eating that uses Love's power instead of willpower to make the change stick.

There is no dieting here—no menus, no amounts, no absolutes. Why should I tell you what to eat on some hypothetical days one through seven as if you had only a week to live? You have a life to live, and it isn't hypothetical. Besides, in real life every day is "day one." At this point in your progress along the continuum of inner to outer well-being, you're ready for recommendations, not regimentation. You don't need rules to resist but tools to get new concepts off the drawing board and into practice.

The Love-powered diet celebrates the abundance of nature. Its basic food groups are:

- Fruits, preferably fresh but also frozen, unsweetened ones
- Vegetables, raw in salads and as crudités but also steamed, sautéed, and baked (potatoes fit here, too)
- Whole grains, such as breads, pastas, and cereal grains like rice and oats
- Legumes, such as dried beans, peas, lentils, and soy foods such as tofu and tempeh

There is also an auxiliary category of rich relatives. These foods are higher in oil content or in natural sugars than the basic foods. They are used in smaller quantities as condiments or garnishes and can supplement the diet of people who need extra calories to maintain their weight. Rich relatives include nuts and seeds (preferably raw and unsalted), olives, avocado, extra-virgin olive oil; dried fruits, fruit juices, all-fruit jam; and sweeteners such as honey, sorghum, and pure maple syrup.

All this translates into meals such as fruit plates, fruit smoothies (luscious blender shakes), crisp salads, vegetable stir-fries, casseroles and chowders, hearty whole-wheat bread and quick loaves like cornbread and banana bread, an assortment of rice and noodle dishes, Boston baked beans, and satisfying soups such as lentil and split pea. The world of ethnic cooking comes alive for Love-powered chefs, too. You can experiment with dishes from:

- The Middle East: pita sandwiches with hummus (chick-pea spread) or baba ghannouj (eggplant dip), tabbouleh (cracked-wheat salad), rice pilafs
- Italy: eggplant dishes, gnocchi, and an endless array of pasta with vegetables and tomato or wine-based sauces
- India: a variety of vegetable curries with tantalizing complementary chutneys, dal (spicy sauces made from lentils or split peas), pungent rice dishes
- Mexico: chili sans carne (meatless), avocado tostadas, bean burritos, taco salad
- Asia: vegetable sushi, spring rolls, tofu-vegetable stir-fries, lo mein

Even traditional American fare like burgers can be prepared using low-fat, vegetarian recipes. You can create wonderful substitutes for familiar foods so you won't think about what you're no longer eating. You can customize what you eat to fit the way you live. (See Eating to Live on page 135 for more details about food selection and preparation and dining out.)

If you don't quite believe that, it's probably because of a single word in the preceding paragraph: vegetarian. It is true that the Love-powered diet, when followed completely, is vegetarian. In fact, because in its purest form it includes no foods of animal origin, it is a total vegetarian, or vegan, plan. Stay with me on this, and let me reassure you that eating solely from the plant kingdom—most of the time or even all of the time—will not change your politics, your religion, or any other part of yourself that the label "vegetarian" doesn't seem to fit. You never need to use the word if you're not comfortable with it, and because the Love-powered diet doesn't require absolute adherence, you can make progress without becoming strictly vegetarian.

In his book *The McDougall Plan for Super Health and Life-Long Weight Loss*, John McDougall, M.D., suggests a low-fat vegan diet but allows healthy people the option of including some other things on occasion as feast foods. This may work for you, too.

Read the following lists of famous vegetarians of the past and present; you'll soon discover that if you do decide to go all the way with this, you'll be in good company.

Some Famous Vegetarians, Past and Present

PHILOSOPHY AND RELIGION

Buddha

Clement of Alexandria

Ralph Waldo Emerson

Stephen Gaskin

J. Krishnamurti

Plato

Pythagoras

Peter Singer

Socrates

Henry David Thoreau

John Wesley

Ellen G. White

LITERATURE AND JOURNALISM

Louisa May Alcott

Laura Huxley

Colman McCarthy

John Milton

Malcolm Muggeridge

George Bernard Shaw

Percy Bysshe Shelley

Isaac Bashevis Singer

Sir Rabindranath Tagore

Leo Tolstoy

SCIENCE AND MEDICINE

Max Bircher-Benner

Deepak Chopra

Charles Darwin

Thomas Edison

Albert Einstein

Sylvester Graham

John Harvey Kellogg

Sir Isaac Newton

Albert Schweitzer

Leonardo da Vinci

POLITICS AND SOCIAL REFORM

Susan B. Anthony
Clara Barton
Annie Besant
General William Booth
Julio Cesar Chávez
Mahatma Gandhi
Horace Greeley
Helen and Scott Nearing

SPORTS

Ridgely Abele (World Championship, karate)
Peter Burwash (Canadian champion and Davis Cup star, tennis)
Andreas Cahling (Mr. International, bodybuilding)
Ruth Heidrich (Ironman triathlete)
Kathy Johnson (Olympic gymnast)
Billie Jean King (tennis champion)
Tony LaRussa (manager, St. Louis Cardinals baseball team)
Carl Lewis (Olympic runner)
Sixto Linares (world record holder, 24-hour triathlon: 4.8 miles
    swimming, 185 miles cycling, 52.5 miles running)
Edwin Moses (Olympic gold medalist, undefeated for eight years in
    400-meter hurdles)
Bess Motta ("20-Minute Workout," aerobics)
Gayle Olinekova (marathoner)
Bill Pearl (four-time Mr. Universe, bodybuilding)
Bill Pickering (world record, swimming the English Channel)
Stan Price (world record, bench press, weight lifting)
Murray Rose (world records for both 400- and 1500-meter freestyle,
    swimming)

ENTERTAINMENT

Rosanna Arquette

Bob Barker

Kim Basinger

Meredith Baxter-Birney

Jeff Beck

Ellen Burstyn

Julie Christie

Elvira

Melissa Etheridge

Peter Gabriel

Boy George

Dick Gregory

Dustin Hoffman

Casey Kasem

K.D. Lang

Cloris Leachman

Annie Lennox

Hayley Mills

Lisa Monet

Paul and Linda McCartney

Kevin Nealon

Olivia Newton-John

Stevie Nicks

Phylicia Rashad

Fred "Mister" Rogers

Ravi Shankar

Sting

Cicely Tyson

Lindsay Wagner

Carl Weathers

Dennis Weaver

Vanessa Williams

Paul Winter

Gretchen Wyler

A TASTE FOR QUALITY
● ● ● ● ● ● ● ● ● ● ● ● ● ● ● ● ● ●

LOVE-POWERED EATING DOESN'T JUST BYPASS ANIMAL FOODS, it leaves out (most of the time) the highly refined, overprocessed phony foods that we're fond of calling junk.

The majority of items found in convenience stores and gas stations, much of what's in an ordinary bakery, and probably everything at the movie theater (unless there's popcorn not popped in coconut oil) is junk food. The super-market has its share of nutritionally vacant items, and some of them can even creep into a health food store. Reading labels is a good practice, but the best food is usually fresh food—no package, no label.

For a Love-powered diet to give you all it can, you'll want to avoid any food that isn't good enough for you—just the way your mother told you not to date Sammy Smith for that very reason. If it's high in sugar (when sugar is near the top of an ingredients list, it's high), high in salt (enough to make you thirsty), or very fatty (if it's fried, "melts in your mouth," or leaves a shine on your napkin), well, meet Sammy Smith.

Everyone knows that junk food is a nutritional disaster, packs in the calories, and causes a yen for more of the same. In addition, it simply isn't becoming to someone who's out to love herself more. You can go to an elegant restaurant and consume a thousand calories in a special dinner with a special person and leave there feeling super about the world and everything that's in it—yourself included. Or you could go to some fast-food place, gobble up a thousand calories in 4.2 minutes, and feel fat and guilty as you toss the wrappers. Cultivate your taste for quality food and select the best food that you can afford.

Go for quality drinks, too, since many are questionable. Alcohol, with its empty calories and mood-altering potential, should be limited to moderate consumption, if you choose to drink at all. A typical soda contains some 9 teaspoons of sugar in a 12-ounce can, and no artificial sweetener has been proven unequivocally safe.

The caffeine in cola as well as in coffee and tea can also be a problem. Caffeine is a stimulant. The easiest way to modify a caffeine-induced buzz is to eat, and many people do this unconsciously. Caffeine can also suppress the appetite temporarily, but it comes back like gangbusters. Dieters usually drink lots of coffee, tea, and cola, and dieters usually relapse. It's possible that there is a caffeine connection.

According to Agatha Thrash, M.D., in her book *Nutrition for Vegetarians*, "Any drug that will stimulate the nerves will stimulate the appetite in susceptible people. This includes coffee, tea, colas, and chocolate. These beverages stimulate cravings."

If you consume beverages that contain caffeine, pay attention to the ways they affect your attitude and your appetite. You may decide to discontinue or moderate your use and try herbal teas, sparkling mineral water, and natural spritzers (mineral water and fruit juice) instead. The drink that helped get a diet-cola hankering the size of Texas off my back is licorice tea. Hot or iced, this herbal drink is naturally sweet but calorically negligible.

With animal products, junk foods, and iffy drinks out of your diet, you will also have inadvertently eliminated all or most of your personal binge foods. You may, however, have others, and it's important that you come to terms with them. Not everyone who wants to lose a few pounds has binge foods, but if you've ever been on an eating binge—that's an all-out eating frenzy that leaves you feeling intoxicated—you're probably intimately acquainted with them. I've heard them described as "better than sex" and "one bite is too many and a thousand aren't enough." These are the foods that encourage appetite instead of extinguishing it. You really can't eat just one. If you have some today, you'll need more tomorrow. In other words, binge foods are addictive.

The usual recipe for a binge food is fat plus sugar or fat plus salt. Common culprits, then, are what you'd expect: ice cream, chips, chocolate, pastries, and cheese. But even something as subtle as combining nuts and raisins for trail mix can turn two otherwise innocuous foods into the makings of some overeater's lost weekend. Besides, binge foods are intensely personal. For a given individual, something about the taste or texture of almost any food, or past associations with it, can make it far more than just something to eat. You may have trouble with a broad category of foods—sugar, meat, flour, or anything at your mom's house—or specific items such as granola, yogurt, dates, peanut butter, or white bread.

If you can be really honest with yourself, you'll probably realize that you already know your own red-light foods. You may not want to claim them, but you may as well—they've already claimed you. If you're unsure about a specific suspect, try to eat a little and save the rest for the following week. If you can't do it, or if you think incessantly about it while it sits in the cupboard or fridge, you have yourself a binge food.

The point in identifying these is to protect yourself from infiltrators out to sabotage your victory. If you had an enemy who was set on harming you, you would do everything in your power to protect yourself. You would notify the police and obtain a restraining order to keep that person away from your house. Understand that any food you haven't been able to eat reasonably since you cut teeth is as threatening to you as that enemy. The safest path to tread with a binge food is the one that leads away from it. In other words, don't eat it—not because I said so, but because you would rather not socialize with a dietary hit man.

The prospect of living without some food you have depended upon can seem unbearable, but you can do it. The secret is to think in terms of today instead of eternity. There is disagreement among eating-disorders experts and recovering overeaters (who are also experts, in my opinion) on whether or not these dynamite foods can ever be defused. That is to say, can the allure of carrot cake come down to that of carrot sticks? I've found that I'm able to eat anything that I choose to eat today providing my spiritual life is in order. Other overeaters in recovery—people every bit as attentive to their spiritual lives as I am—assiduously avoid certain foods, usually sweets.

With what the Twelve Step programs call HOW—honesty, openmindedness, and willingness—you'll find your own way with binge foods. They are potentially loaded weapons, but they will in time lose much of their attraction. One of these days, you'll find yourself looking at a onetime temptation as if it were an old flame and thinking, "What did I ever see in that one?"

Snacking—with wild abandon at least—can meet a similar fate. With the Love-powered diet, you can elect to snack on something that will support your health, or you may decide not to snack. Every so often, some study reports that eating small, frequent meals (snacking or "grazing") is superior to having three regular meals. This works for certain people and there are, in fact, medical conditions that require it. For most of us, though, the sanest approach is also the simplest: three reasonable meals a day, eaten on a fairly predictable schedule.

In the earliest stages of your lifestyle change, you may need large meals to bridge the gap between binge eating and moderation. That's fine. Begin wherever you can. With a commitment to three meals, you'll find that, in starting to eat only three times, you'll have to stop only three times. For anyone with a food problem, stopping is the hard part. Moreover, society is set up for three meals a day. You go on vacation and stay at a bed-and-breakfast. Your workday is punctuated with a lunch hour. You're invited out for dinner.

As you embark on this adventure, you'll be enjoying bountiful meals and may well find that eating three of these a day with nothing but living in between is fully adequate. On the other hand, this is a low-fat food plan that includes lots of water-rich fruits and vegetables that are efficiently processed by your digestive apparatus. They don't stay with you like heavy, fatty foods that must be laboriously digested. Therefore, you may well want something to eat at morning break time, mid-afternoon, or before bed.

The best snack is a piece of fruit. This is the original, portable fast food.

The natural sugars in fruit will pick up your energy, and it's as close to fat-free as you're going to get. Have fruit between meals if you want it. Raw vegetables make good snacks, too, although they can seem too much like diet food for some. In any event, you never have to go hungry. You may at times choose to feel hungry; and that's all right, too. Oh, I know that no book like this is supposed to suggest that you'll ever feel any less satiated than a just-nursed infant, but that isn't realistic. Mom doesn't pack us lunches anymore, and there will be times when we would like to eat and will need to wait. Saying no sometimes is as much a part of the privilege of adulthood as saying yes.

This is where flexibility comes in, flexibility of your food plan and of your thinking. When we are spiritually fit, we can make rational decisions, even when those decisions are about food. Let's say that you have to dash to the airport without having supper, and the kiosk near your flight gate only has candy bars and salted peanuts. You have a choice. You can buy a candy bar or some peanuts, or you can choose to feel a little hungry and wait until food that's healthier is available. What would you do? If it were me, I would go without for the time being if dinner were going to be served on the plane. If, however, I had to wait until I got to Cincinnati for my next meal, I would get a bag of peanuts. Even though I don't usually eat salted nuts and generally stick with fruit between meals, this would be a perfectly legitimate action in a less-than-perfect situation.

There may be some fabled diet land where airport newsstands sell celery and where you can have half a banana today and the other half won't turn brown while you save it for the following day. I just don't live in a place like that, and you don't either. Around here, it makes more sense to have a whole banana and maybe some peanuts every once in a while. You can do that with Love-powered eating because it's designed to work in the real world, the same world that actively benefits when you choose Love-powered foods. This brings us back to those five points that we came up with at the beginning of this chapter.

A Love-powered diet is generous, delicious, and aesthetically pleasing.

A downside of dieting is lack of food. You're told to compensate by using a smaller plate. Now you can use a standard plate and a big salad bowl. If a substantial salad with light, no-oil dressing is the center of your meal, ordinary salad bowls are a joke. Uncooked vegetables as well as fruits are both low in fat and high in water; therefore they are low in calories. The filling starches from which you'll make most of your entrées—rice, pasta, beans, potatoes (yes, plural!)—are low-fat foods as well, so they're lower in calories than traditional main dishes.

In addition, some evidence suggests that calories from fat are more fattening than the same number of calories from carbohydrates. And even the leaner animal foods are generally fattier than grains, vegetables, and most beans.

I'm not suggesting that because most Love-powered foods won't put you at odds with the bathroom scale, you should overeat. The latest resurgence of high-protein diets came in response to widespread pig-outs on carbohydrates—usually refined flour and sugar products, which I'm not recommending anyway. I am saying, however, that the concept of a moderate portion has to be redefined when you adopt a low-fat diet. If you're having salad, steamed asparagus, and corn on the cob for dinner, don't have an ear of corn: Have three or four and a roll, too. And those boxes of rice pilaf don't serve six anymore. They served six with roast beef. As a main course, they'll serve two or three.

Not only are Love-powered portions generous, the variety of foods from which you'll choose is enormous. When people find out that you're doing this, they'll say, "But what do you eat?" Take it from me: They wouldn't stand still long enough to hear all the marvelous foods on nature's table. (See Eating to Live on page 135 for lists of some of the many foods you'll enjoy.) When you're eating natural foods and concentrating on those from the plant kingdom, you'll become far more aware of seasonal fruits and vegetables. As you travel, you'll find regional delights that are lost to people on the burger-and-fries circuit. There are hundreds of varieties of vegetables and fruits, dozens of kinds of grains and legumes, and plenty of interesting specialty and convenience foods made from them.

From this abundance, you can select what you like. You don't have to eat any specific food—not grapefruit, not spinach, not soybeans. You build your eating plan around foods you already like, and with a little daring you can discover both delicious new foods and tasty new ways to fix old favorites.

Either way, what you'll offer yourself and others to eat will look beautiful. A supermarket checker once bagged my week's provisions and said, "I've had this job for 15 years and I've never seen such pretty groceries!" That's because fruits and vegetables really are edible works of art, and whether in a shopping cart or on a serving tray, they are very appealing to people. Natural, vegetarian foods entice the eye and have wonderful fragrances and distinctive flavors. They tantalize several senses, and meals based on them invite appreciation and the slower pace that's essential in retraining eating habits. It's also pleasant to be in the company of these foods. If you were going to meet a friend in the city, wouldn't you rather rendezvous at a fruit stand than at a butcher shop or fish market? And if you went back to your place for the kind of simple but elegant dinner you will soon be adept at preparing, cleanup would be a breeze. Greasy pots do not exist when you don't fix greasy foods, and that counts as aesthetically pleasing, too.

A Love-powered diet promotes high-level health as well as normal weight.

"I have lived quite long enough and am trying to die," wrote vegetarian George Bernard Shaw at 84, "but I simply cannot do it. A single beefsteak would finish me, but I cannot bring myself to swallow it. I am oppressed with a dread of living forever. That is the only disadvantage of vegetarianism."

There isn't any diet, of course, that can substitute for genes programmed for longevity, but a poor diet can keep you from reaching your potential for both quality and length of life. (For more on the many health benefits of low-fat, minimally processed plant foods, see page 117.) Here are statistics reported by John Robbins in his book *Diet for a New America* and taken here from the EarthSave booklet "Realities for the 90s."

- The average American man has a 50 percent chance of dying from a heart attack; the average total vegetarian man reduces that risk to 4 percent.
- No country in the world with a high intake of meat has a low incidence of colon cancer.
- Women who eat eggs three or more days a week, compared to less than once a week, have a three times greater risk of developing fatal ovarian cancer.
- Men who consume meats, dairy products, and eggs daily, as compared to sparingly, run a 3.6 times greater risk of developing fatal prostate cancer.
- The average measurable bone loss of female meat-eaters at age 65 is 35 percent; in vegetarian women it is 18 percent.

A variety of factors may account for the apparent superiority of a vegetarian or near-vegetarian diet. In replacing animal foods with unrefined grains, fruits, vegetables, and legumes, a dietary program results that is:

- Cholesterol-free (cholesterol in our diets comes only from foods of animal origin)
- Low in fats, especially saturated fats
- High in natural carbohydrates
- Rich in fiber
- Abundant in vitamins A and C, which some research indicates may protect against certain cancers, and other possible anticarcinogens such as indoles in cruciferous (cabbage family) vegetables and protease inhibitors in legumes
- Adequate but not excessive in protein (too much protein has been linked with osteoporosis, kidney stones, and deterioration of kidney function)
- Markedly lower in pesticide residues, particularly chlorinated hydrocarbons, which accumulate in our body fat
- Bulky and satisfying to assuage hunger without excess calories

It is, therefore, widely accepted in medical literature that vegans, people who eat only plant foods and no meat, fish, eggs, or dairy products, typically weigh 8 to 20 pounds less than omnivores, eaters of both plants and animals. The omnivores average 17 to 22 pounds over ideal weight. The serendipitous thing about vegans and weight is that their slimness is not something they work at. It happens naturally—without hunger, suffering, or willpower. That's precisely how it will happen for you, provided that you practice the spiritual principles that will keep you from needing to eat for a fix and build your diet predominantly from the four Love-powered food groups.

A Love-powered diet is economical and provides plenty for everybody.

You can afford a Love-powered diet, even if you're a full-time student, a retired person on a fixed income, or a food-stamp recipient. The staples for this eating style are among the most inexpensive foods in the marketplace: rice, beans, whole-wheat flour and bread, potatoes, carrots, greens and other seasonal vegetables, apples, oranges, bananas, and other fruits selected when they're most abundant and least costly. You'll be saving cash by skipping the high-ticket items like meat and cheese—as well as the junk foods, which may sometimes be bargains until you consider the physiological price you pay for them.

You certainly can spend money on rare, tropical fruits, exotic vegetables (I'm astounded by how many vegetables come in purple), health food store convenience items, and gourmet specialties. You don't need these, though, to design Love-powered menus that are nutritious and conducive to bringing your best body into being. Simple foods—those that the Earth provides generously for all—can be the makings of elegant repasts, celebrations of life and health in good taste and good conscience.

A Love-powered diet respects all life.

In summer and fall, the classifieds are filled with ads for "pick-your-own" places, inviting city folks on a country outing that will bring in a miniature harvest of apples or berries. That's the same time of year that the gardeners are out in force, turning suburban yards into small truck farms or greening midtown balconies with lettuce and radish and tomato plants. People delight in these pursuits, even before the fruits of their labors reach the dinner table.

Throughout the year, however, something else is going on. Animals are being slaughtered for meat, not a few but nearly 6 billion a year in the United States alone. We usually don't stop to think that a Kansas City steak was recently a Kansas cow, but as philosopher Peter Singer wrote in his book *Animal Liberation*, "For most humans, especially those in modern urban and suburban communities, the most direct form of contact with nonhuman animals is at mealtime: We eat them."

Many people believe that this is just as it should be and it certainly isn't my place to meddle in your personal ethics. You need not be a vegetarian to develop the spiritual connection that will free you from the need to abuse food. Maintaining that connection does, however, ask that we take responsibility for our actions. Would you, in an ordinary, nonemergency situation, kill an animal and eat it? Most people find the prospect repugnant—quite unlike picking apples or growing tomato plants.

In fact, most people I know support the killing of animals for meat through the food choices they make yet refuse to tour a slaughterhouse. I asked 15 of them, and none would go. I went by myself. There was a particular cow I will always remember. She was old, a reject from a dairy herd; "used up," the man said. She seemed used to people and trusting, so she didn't require the cattle prod—an instrument that is capable of producing first-degree burns—to walk the ramp to the metal enclosure where she would be stunned with the captive bolt pistol. When the worker came at her with the stunner, she crouched to avoid it. He whistled at her, the way I imagined he might whistle at his dog when he got home that evening. She raised her head in response and was shot with the captive bolt. She dropped to the floor and within minutes was unceremoniously transformed from a being to beef. "You have just dined," wrote Ralph Waldo Emerson, "and however scrupulously the slaughterhouse is concealed in the distance of miles, there is complicity."

Unlike in Emerson's day, though, there is a problem in the barnyard as well as at the slaughterhouse. Most of the animals raised for food today come from factory farms where they may be confined to small cages or stalls, and are dehorned, detailed, debeaked, and mutilated in other ways. Many are denied exercise, companionship, natural diets, and other basic needs, and there are no federal laws protecting them.

Consideration for the animals involved may never be your motivation for a diet that excludes animal foods. Still, expect that as you adopt some of the principles found here your overall reverence for life will expand. You may not interpret or express that reverence in the way that someone else might, but expect to see it in your life because it will be there. As psychologist Virginia Satir wrote, "Spiritual power can be seen in a person's reverence for life—hers and all others, including animals and nature, with a recognition of a universal life force referred to by many as God."

A Love-powered diet is environmentally sustainable.

It is as gentle to the Earth as it is to animals and arteries. Eating low on the food chain (following the Love-powered diet or one similar to it) can be just as

easy to incorporate into an ecologically aware lifestyle as other responsible practices like recycling cans and recharging batteries.

Why a diet that does not depend on animal foods is vital in restoring health
to an ailing planet is explained in the following facts and figures from Robbins.

About 75 percent of U.S. topsoil has been lost to date, and 85 percent of
U.S. topsoil loss is directly associated with livestock raising.

Some 260 million acres of U.S. forests have been cleared for cropland to
produce a meat-centered diet.

Every individual who switches to a complete vegetarian diet saves an acre
of trees each year.

About 33 percent of all raw materials (base products of farming, forestry,
and mining, including fossil fuels) consumed by the United States are devoted to the production of livestock.

More than half the water used for all purposes in the United States goes
for livestock production.

Livestock in this country produce 230,000 pounds of excrement every second. Feedlots do not have sewage systems, so with every rainstorm a part
of the one billion tons of waste generated annually in confinement opera-
tions goes into streams, rivers, and groundwater.

To get a single calorie of protein from beef requires 78 calories of fossil fuel.
One calorie of protein from soybeans requires just 2 calories of fossil fuel.

Statistics can be numbing and the whole notion of an environmental crisis can seem so overwhelming that the very thought of it can push a shut-off
valve in our psyches to divert our thinking elsewhere. True, the Earth's ills are
enormous and it will take action on myriad fronts to heal them. Contributing to
the well-being of the planet with Earth-loving food choices is one such action,
one which takes no time and no extraordinary effort. You're probably busy with

all sorts of things, but you will stop for lunch—making it a Love-powered meal can be an effortless donation to a most deserving planet.

In addition to the environmental benefits brought about by eating low on the food chain, there are subtler ways in which simpler eating supports an eco-ethic. Since you'll be selecting natural foods, many of which can be bought in bulk and put in reusable containers, you'll be using fewer packaging materials. You'll be less likely to visit fast-food places with their plethora of disposables, and since you won't have meat scraps, all of your garbage can be composted if you're so inclined. With the money you save, you can buy some food that is organically grown, and with more fresh fruits and salads in your diet, you may use your stove less often and save energy. Also, this is clean eating; you will have fewer dishes to wash so you'll use less detergent and hot water.

A Love-powered diet may cause the environmentalist within you to emerge by inviting nature into your kitchen. Don't be surprised if you find yourself growing parsley and chives in clay pots on your windowsills or raising a crop of alfalfa sprouts on your counter. You might even find yourself planting a tree that, in a few years or several, will bear fruit or nuts. When this was first suggested to me, I argued, "Why should I plant a fruit tree? I won't even be living in this house when it gets its first peach." But "someone will be living there," I was reminded. A tree, then, can be a contribution to strangers and the Earth. And eating from trees, gardens, and fields can be a gift to yourself, one of all sorts of ways that you'll discover to make the Love in your life practical and viable.

• •

NOURISHED BY LOVE

Choose natural foods from the plant kingdom—fruits, vegetables, whole grains, and legumes. If you don't want to be a complete vegetarian, use animal foods more for variety and flavor than as major players.

Know that plant foods may be eaten generously. Have ample portions from the four food groups discussed earlier. If you enjoy salad, eat all you want as long as you're not using a rich, oily dressing. (In that case, replace or limit the dressing, not the salad.)

Avoid second helpings as a general rule. When you serve yourself, start with enough. If someone serves you a piddling portion, have more.

Rethink the main course. Make sure that rice, potatoes, or a large salad with pasta or beans in it can fit there. Round out meals with more vegetables, bread, and so forth.

Use rich relatives, like nuts, avocado, and dried fruit, sparingly. (If you're healthy and don't need to lose weight or can handle the extra calories, you can eat more of these.)

Go for quality. You deserve better than junk food. For the most part, leave sugar, grease, and excess salt on their side of the tracks—the wrong side. Caffeine and alcohol consumption should be reduced or eliminated.

Have three meals a day unless your doctor wants you to eat more often. Sit down during meals. Have a place setting. Try not to rush through it.

If you want a snack, have fruit. Feeling hungry for a while before a meal is okay, too. Unless you have a medical condition like diabetes or hypoglycemia that requires you to eat small, frequent meals, your choosing to go without food between lunch and dinner and between dinner and bedtime will not harm you.

Eat only when you're emotionally and spiritually centered. If you feel that you're about to eat for a fix, even at mealtime, get yourself together first by calling a supportive friend, taking a walk, or writing in your journal.

Avoid personal binge foods. These are the foods that seem to incite overeating or that you obsess over when they're around. A Love-powered diet eliminates most of the common ones, but recognize and respect yours.

Leave a little food on your plate. I've heard it called the angel bite. You're not a failure when you don't do this, but you get lots of inner nourishment when you do.

Follow the "Nutritional Guidelines" below. Familiarize yourself with the fundamental nutritional information in Healthy and Whole on page 111, and help ensure your general health with the suggestions in Love-Yourself Living on page 198.

Give less power to the scale. Find a sensible midpoint between frequent weighing and refusing to find out what you weigh. Decide on weighing yourself once or twice a month and stay with that. You will lose weight. Give yourself an edge with exercise. If you have a history of crash dieting, or if you have been bulimic, it may take time for your body to respond to normal, healthful eating with the loss of weight you're looking for. Be patient. Concentrate on self-acceptance and on enjoying the day at hand. Remember that you're working with the laws of nature. They can't be rushed and they can't be cheated. Allow yourself to be a part of the natural process. This is for life, so there's no reason to hurry. Don't be discouraged by a slow-moving scale. If you want to be impressed by a number, look at your Love-powered cholesterol level.

Get the help you need. Continue to ask God or your Higher Power each morning for help in eating reasonably that day. Say thanks at night, even if your eating wasn't perfect. Attend Overeaters Anonymous. Read the books listed in Suggested Reading on page 237.

Give yourself priority status. Allow yourself time for meals and food preparation, for meditation, exercise, support group meetings, and whatever else you need. Remember that this isn't selfishness—it's self-preservation.

NUTRITIONAL GUIDELINES

THE LOVE-POWERED DIET PROVIDES OPTIMUM NUTRITION for your health. Following these guidelines will further ensure that. If you are under a doctor's care, consult him about your eating plan.

If you are pregnant or nursing, follow the advice of your health care provider. For additional information, read *Pregnancy, Children, and the Vegan Diet* by Michael Klaper, M.D., available from the American Vegan Society, or *The Vegan Diet during Pregnancy, Lactation, and Childhood* by Reed Mangels, R.D., Ph.D., available from the Vegetarian Resource Group. For addresses to write to these organizations, see Some Helpful Organizations on page 241.

1. Eat from all four Love-powered food groups daily: vegetables, fruits, whole grains, and legumes. If you wish to use animal products, do so in moderation.

2. Have at least one large salad every day and include in it a variety of leafy greens (romaine, leaf lettuce, spinach) plus other vegetables.

3. Include foods rich in vitamin C such as citrus fruits, cantaloupe, bell peppers, tomatoes, and strawberries.

4. Eat foods with a high vitamin C content along with iron-rich foods. This helps increase iron absorption by your body. High-iron foods include beans, peas, and lentils; dried fruit such as prunes and figs; almonds and cashews; whole grains; and leafy greens (the greens come with their own vitamin C as well).

5. Include at least two daily servings of calcium-rich foods such as collards, kale, broccoli, oatmeal, soybeans, tofu cultured with calcium sulfate, almonds, calcium-fortified orange juice, or calcium-fortified soy milk or rice milk (at health food stores). Virtually all your food will provide some calcium, and much research indicates that people need less of this mineral on a plant-based diet than on one high in animal protein.

6. Be sure to get vitamin D through moderate exposure to sunlight. This is of particular concern to dark-skinned people living in northern latitudes.

7. Supplement your diet regularly with a source of vitamin B_{12} (cobalamin) to meet the Daily Value of 6 micrograms if you haven't eaten animal products for three years or if you are pregnant or nursing. B_{12} tablets contain more than this and may be taken weekly. Many vegetarian foods are fortified with B_{12}, including some meat analogs, nutritional yeasts, some brands of fortified soy milk, and some commonly available cereals, such as Nutri-Grain and Kellogg's Bran Flakes. (For more on vitamin B_{12}, see page 125.)

8. Eat a vegetable from the cabbage family (broccoli, brussels sprouts, cauliflower) at least four times a week.

9. Don't overdo protein by eating too many beans—a cup a day is plenty. The Love-powered diet will keep your protein intake at the proper level. Provided you obtain adequate calories from a variety of natural foods, you will secure ample protein without special foods or food combinations.

10. Be moderate in your use of nuts, seeds, olives, and avocado and be ever so sparing in your use of oil for cooking and in salad dressings to keep fat consumption low. Cut down by water-sautéing, substituting applesauce for shortening in baking, and using no-stick cookware. (For more information on low-fat recipe substitutions, see "Fat Zappers" on page 177.) Even so, if you eat a total vegetarian diet, your diet will automatically be low in total fat and very low in artery-clogging saturated fat without your having to be excessively concerned.

SEVEN
Healthy and Whole

THIS IS A TECHNOLOGY ALERT. BY THAT I MEAN THAT THE UPCOMING chapter is fairly detailed in its discussion of nutrition and health as they relate to low-fat vegetarian eating. This important information can help you confidently make this change, plan meals that will best support your health, and answer the questions you're sure to be asked when people see that you are eating differently. You may want to share this chapter with your doctor or nutritionist, but if you're not up for facts and figures right now, feel free to skip ahead and come back to this later.

People are very trusting about nutrition. Oh, we can sound pretty sophisticated while talking about amino acids and polyunsaturates. Even so, don't you think most people believe that anything on a grocer's shelf that doesn't have a skull and crossbones on it is, if not a full-fledged health food, at least quite suitable for human consumption? Most folks pride themselves on being omnivorous. "I can eat anything" and "I have a cast-iron stomach" are boastful statements. Nevertheless, the results of eating everything edible and treating our stomachs as if they were indeed formed in a smelter are devastating.

We see these results in overweight, digestive disorders, and degenerative diseases. What's more, this seems normal. Repeated diets, popping antacids, even submitting to major surgery are practices so common they're regarded as inevitable. This simpler way of eating, although not a panacea, may be an alternative. When introduced to it, however, people often respond defensively. They want to know, "Where do you get your protein? Where do you get your calcium? Where do you get your iron?" The answer is that all these nutrients come to us from the plant kingdom. By eating plant foods, we get them directly. With animal foods, we get them secondhand.

Still, most people eat everything and assume that doing so is essential for good health. That assumption has been substantiated over the years with the assorted caveats applied to vegetarian diets. These include such assertions as: "It's all right not to eat meat, but you need to have plenty of milk and eggs and maybe some fish every so often"; and "Vegetarians need to take lots of supplements and add to their meals things such as protein powder, bonemeal, and cod-liver oil"; and "You can only eat that way if you combine your food just right and plan every meal very carefully."

I'll bet even skydivers and hang-glider pilots don't get such persistent warnings. To top it off, not one of these arguments has an actual basis in current scientific information. On the contrary, natural vegetarian foods are generally rich in nutritional value, largely low in fat, and absolutely free of cholesterol, so a lot of the "balancing" that we think of as necessary in designing any food plan is taken care of with this simple choice.

This is one important reason why this eating style can be a helpful tool for keeping food obsession from resurfacing: You don't have to spend an inordinate amount of time thinking about your food. Natural vegetarian meals are complete and nourishing. Your body knows what to do with them so you can stop counting, quantifying, measuring, and worrying about what you eat. You can put your mind on other things.

WHAT'S SO SAD ABOUT THE STANDARD AMERICAN DIET?

THE PRESTIGIOUS JOURNALS of medicine and nutrition have for decades been dotted with reports connecting the way people eat with many of the ills they endure. A great many of these studies show that vegetarian or near-vegetarian diets can reduce the risk for many of the diseases and disorders that plague modern society. Apparently, several key differences exist between a natural vegetarian diet and the standard American diet. A way of eating based on plant foods is naturally low in fat, high in fiber, and moderate in protein. The typical American diet, on the other hand, is built around animal foods, is high in fat, deficient in fiber, and excessive in protein.

Animal Foods

In his book *Vegan Nutrition: Pure and Simple*, Michael Klaper, M.D., makes the following straightforward declaration: "The body of *Homo sapiens* has no nutritional requirement for the flesh of animals, for the eggs of chickens, or for the milk of cows." Not only can we be well-nourished without them, there is ample evidence that such foods are actually harmful. In addition to the overload of cholesterol, fat, and protein in most of them and their dearth of fiber, animal foods are also the major dietary source of purines, which cause a rise in fat and glucose levels in the blood—a rise likely to encourage fat storage in the body. Meats are deficient in carbohydrates, the food component that should account for 60 to 80 percent of the calories ingested. (Carbohydrate-deficient diets lead to decreased endurance.)

Because the levels of toxins in animal foods are much higher than those in plants (in some studies, 16 times higher), eating plants instead of animals greatly reduces our intake of these poisons. Of course, choosing organic produce can also result in a marked decrease in the amount of synthetic pesticides we consume. Even so, it is believed that the average person consumes far more of these in animal foods than in vegetable foods.

And pesticide residues aren't the only extras in a slab of steak or bucket of chicken. Growth hormones are commonly used in livestock production, and 55 percent of the antibiotics used in the United States are routinely fed to animals on farms. It is, however, believed to have contributed to the noticeable rise in antibiotic-resistant infections over the past 30 years. Stress hormones secreted by the animal prior to slaughter also become a part of the meat.

Fish, too, although not intentionally fed potential toxins by humans, are subject to the effects of chemical runoff in our rivers, lakes, and seas. Although many people who are otherwise vegetarian choose to include some fish in their diets and do so successfully, it is nevertheless a fact that many fish show serious concentrations of heavy metals, mutation-inducing hydrocarbons, and radioactivity from nuclear pollution.

High in Fat
....

The typical Western diet with its reliance on meats, fish, eggs, and dairy products, along with fried foods and rich baked goods, provides too much fat— 36 percent of calories on average—as well as artery-clogging cholesterol. Fats carry calories at more than double the amount of either proteins or carbohydrates (9 calories per gram for fat, 4 for proteins and carbohydrates). In other words, eating fat means getting more calories from less food. Eating enough high-fat foods to feel full is likely to lead to weight gain, but cutting portion sizes to include these foods results in leaving the table hungry—the first step in the demise of one more diet.

Because the media likes new and revolutionary ideas, it had a great run with low-fat foods when the health problems with diets high in fat began to surface. Once low-fat was no longer hot, the trend swung back to recommendations for more protein in the diet and a loosening up on concern about fat. Trends aside, human physiology didn't just happen to change. It's as difficult for the body to deal with an onslaught of fat—and, for that matter, with too much protein—as it ever was.

It is true that when low-fat and fat-free foods became a cash cow for food manufacturers, lots of people went in for orgies of overeating on concentrated sweets and other manufactured products simply because the packages proclaimed a fat-free status. Some people ate so many fat-free cookies and crackers and cakes that they actually gained weight. This kind of foolishness does not negate the basic reality that excess fat is harmful to health and that a low-fat diet based on real food—not mass-produced junk food, whether high or low in fat—is ideal.

Not only do fats have more calories than other foods, the body likes to hang on to calories from fat. It's a physiological principle that many of the excess calories from carbohydrates are stored in the liver as glycogen so they can be drawn upon for use as energy. According to John McDougall, M.D., author of *The McDougall Plan for Super Health and Life-Long Weight Loss*, fats ingested in foods can be appropriated for body fat much more easily.

Animal foods have, as a rule, a much higher fat content than do vegetables, fruits, grains, and legumes. In addition, animal fats are of a different type than vegetable fats. They are primarily saturated, and it is saturated fat that plays a part in elevating blood cholesterol levels. A few plant foods—primarily coconut, chocolate, and palm oil—are also high in saturated fat.

Cholesterol itself is not found in any plant food; it's made in the livers of animals, including humans. We make all we need. The cholesterol obtained from food is extra and accounts in part for the abnormally high blood cholesterol levels prevalent in this country. While numerous studies have associated elevated cholesterol levels with heart disease, a low blood cholesterol level may be a reasonable indicator of protection against other degenerative conditions as well.

The higher the plasma cholesterol level, the higher is the risk for so-called diseases of affluence: cancers, heart disease, diabetes—the kinds of disease we see in the West, says T. Colin Campbell, Ph.D., a key researcher in the Cornell-China-Oxford Project on Nutrition, Health, and Environment, the largest population study of diet and health ever conducted. "This is pretty remarkable," says Dr. Campbell, "because the plasma cholesterol levels in China are roughly between 100 and 200 milligrams per deciliter. In other words, their high is our low. What this is really saying in a sense is the lower the cholesterol level, the better. High cholesterol levels are related to the consumption of animal foods, and it apparently doesn't take very much of them."

Even the so-called lean cuts of meat have significant levels of saturated fat plus cholesterol. Eating poultry is only a slight improvement and some fish can be extremely high in cholesterol, even though most fish is lower in fat content than meat. There are some vegetable foods that are high in fat—oils, margarine, nuts, seeds, olives, avocadoes, and, to a lesser degree, full-fat soybean products—but the fat in these foods is primarily unsaturated. These fats have not been implicated in heart disease as have the saturated fats prevalent in animal foods, but it's wise to avoid an excess of all fats. (Both saturated and unsaturated fats have the same high caloric density.)

Love-powered eating outshines the American diet in that the latter gives high-fat foods such as meat and eggs star billing at meals. Milk, eggs, butter, and cheese are also used in preparing other foods from side dishes to desserts, and high-fat vegetable foods, like salad and cooking oils, margarine, and peanut butter, are used as well. A pure Love-powered diet eliminates cholesterol and most saturated fat, so the majority of people can enjoy moderate use of the richer plant foods without difficulty. If you don't plan to be a purist—and for the purpose of getting your body in shape and healing your relationship with food, you don't have to be—remember that animal foods count as rich foods, too.

Deficient in Fiber

Meat and dairy products are devoid of the plant fiber required for normal peristaltic action of the colon. In addition, the refining of grains removes most of their fiber content. The upshot of all this is that difficulties in digestion and elimination are so common in "well-fed" societies that bran flakes, fiber-enriched breads, and natural fiber laxatives are common as well. But fiber shouldn't have to be added to the diet. It ought to be there already.

High-fiber diets help lower cholesterol by trapping bile acids in the intestinal tract and allowing them to be excreted, and such a diet is believed to protect against varicose veins, hemorrhoids, hiatus hernia, appendicitis, and gallstones, as well as constipation. The richest sources of fiber are whole grains and legumes; vegetables and fruits are fiber-filled as well.

Excessive in Protein

Periodically, high-protein diets become a sort of buzzword for good nutrition, but we shouldn't be misled on this one. Protein is certainly necessary, but most people get far too much of it and that can be a problem. No more than 15 percent of calories in a normal diet should come from protein, but Americans routinely eat animal foods that contain 41 percent (skim milk, turkey), 79 percent (cottage cheese), and even 88 percent (water-packed tuna) protein.

Although you may have heard that protein burns fat, this assertion is based on the disease state of ketosis that occurs when you consume a risky diet of virtually only protein and fat, with no carbohydrate. In actuality, it is more likely that a high intake of protein—especially that from animal sources—may lead to overweight. In the China health study, it was learned that the Chinese consume, on average, 20 percent more calories per pound of body weight than do Americans, but the Chinese are lighter and leaner than we are by some 25 percent. Part of the reason for this is their level of physical exercise. (When I was in China, I saw bicycles carrying three adults and transporting pieces of furniture as if the bikes were two-wheeled moving vans.) But Campbell believes that their low-protein intake (low in animal protein in particular) may play a part as well.

"It turns out that when one is on a low intake of animal protein, a higher proportion of the energy consumed is actually burned off as heat and it is not laid down as body fat," Campbell explains. "So a low-protein diet, which is characteristic of a vegetarian type of diet, allows obviously more energy to be consumed without running the risk of getting fat from that extra energy—those extra calories. This is an old observation incidentally. It has been around for many, many years, although it has really been much ignored. It's clear that if you look at vegans (true vegetarians that eat only plant foods—no meats or dairy products) in this country, they tend to be rather lean. They tend not to have obesity problems."

Excess protein intake also causes the liver and kidneys to work harder, and it increases the excretion of calcium (see "Calcium or Cowcium?" on page 123).

DISEASE PREVENTION AND THE VEGETARIAN EDGE
• •

F I TELL YOU THAT THE PROOF of all this is in the pudding, you could tell me that I'm using a food addict's favorite phrase, but there *is* absolute truth in it. Following are some of the many ways in which vegetarians are generally better off than omnivores (meat and plant eaters).

Blood pressure. Studies repeatedly show that a low-fat vegetarian diet tends to produce lower blood pressure. This could be due to the trimness of vegetarians, but they also show markedly lower blood viscosity (thickness). The hormonal factors present in meat may also play a role. "Stress hormones are present in an animal at the time of slaughter. The same hormones that cause animals' blood pressures to rise cause ours to rise. It just takes a few molecules," explains George Eisman, R.D., author of *The Most Noble Diet: Food Selection and Ethics.*

Breast cancer. Women who eat meat daily (compared to those who eat it less than once a week) increase their risk of developing breast cancer 3.8 times. Those who eat eggs daily (compared to once a week) increase their risk of breast cancer 2.8 times. Factors accounting for this may include the way in which vegetarian women process estrogen, retaining less of it in their bodies than their meat-eater counterparts, and the later onset of menses in the females of more vegetarian populations.

Diabetes. The decreased chance of obesity in vegans puts them at lower risk for developing Type II (adult-onset) diabetes. Further, according to *Reversing Diabetes* author Julian Whitaker, M.D., "a high-fat diet, even if it doesn't lead to obesity, may bring on diabetes in genetically predisposed individuals—perhaps because the cells of the body are so clogged with fat that they don't receive the insulin message to remove sugar from the bloodstream. The sugar (glucose) accumulates in the blood with disastrous results."

Low-fat diets high in unrefined carbohydrates have clinical application in treating diabetes. Administered under a physician's care, such diets frequently result in the elimination of medication (insulin or oral hypoglycemic agents) in adult-onset diabetes and a reduction in insulin as well as better general control for those with juvenile diabetes.

Heart disease. Vegans have very low cholesterol levels and a concurrently low incidence of heart disease. This finding is not new. Back in June of 1961, an editorial in the *Journal of the American Medical Association* stated that a total vegetarian diet "could prevent 90 percent of our thromboembolic diseases and 97 percent of our coronary occlusions." It was only in the late 1980s, however, that the work of Dean Ornish, M.D., and his colleagues at the University of California at San Francisco confirmed that coronary artery disease can be not only prevented but reversed with a low-fat, vegetarian diet in combination with lifestyle modification including exercise and stress-management techniques.

Obesity. Vegetarians who consume milk and eggs tend to be slightly leaner than the average American, but vegans—people whose diets resemble a total Love-powered diet—are almost always lean.

Osteoporosis. The brittle-bone disease that primarily affects post-menopausal women is less likely to occur among vegetarians because they do not have the high intake of protein that causes calcium to be leached from the bones. Adequate but modest protein consumption combined with regular weight-bearing exercise appears to be the best defense against osteoporosis. Supplementary calcium has not been conclusively proven effective, and when extra calcium is taken in the form of dairy products, any possible benefit from the calcium may be offset by the additional protein in the milk or cheese.

Other diseases. Some other cancers, including those of the ovaries, prostate, colon, and rectum, are statistically less common among vegetarians. Eliminating or drastically reducing meat consumption is standard in the treatment of gout (the purines in meat seem to be the aggravating factor here) and impaired kidney function (in this case, intake of all high-protein foods is curtailed). Studies have shown vegetarians to have a decreased incidence of gallstones, kidney stones, diverticulosis (an intestinal disorder), and stroke. Stroke is the obstruction of an artery to the brain. When an artery to the heart is completely blocked, a heart attack occurs. The same condition—saturated fat and cholesterol impeding blood flow—can account for either. It's merely a matter of location.

This information should tell us that switching to a Love-powered diet is the smartest move we can take in terms of eating habits to provide the best odds for a long, healthy, and enjoyable life. It would make sense that the same food program that protects against so many diseases and lacks so many of the components shown to be harmful to human health would also provide us with what we require nutritionally. According to the dietary guidelines for Americans, we should:

- Eat a variety of foods
- Maintain a healthy weight
- Choose a diet low in total fat, saturated fat, and cholesterol
- Choose a diet with plenty of vegetables, fruits, and grain products
- Use sugars only in moderation
- Use salt and sodium only in moderation
- Avoid alcoholic beverages or keep consumption moderate

These guidelines are reflected in the U.S. Department of Agriculture's Food Guide Pyramid with grains as its broad base, implying that these should form the bulk of a healthful diet. The next tier of the pyramid is vegetables, then fruits, then dairy products as the pyramid narrows, followed by the protein group including animal and vegetable sources of concentrated protein, and finally the tip of the pyramid, which is the fats and sweets to be used sparingly. It's easy to use the pyramid as a guideline and be a partial or total vegetarian if you use other calcium-rich foods (like leafy greens and fortified soy milk) to replace dairy products and vegetable protein (like beans and tofu) to replace meat and, if you like, to replace eggs and cheese, too.

THE NEW FOUR FOOD GROUPS

The Physicians Committee for Responsible Medicine has its own plan that works for vegetarians without making substitutions. Following are the "New Four Food Groups" and the foods you can eat to get your fill from each.

Whole grains. This group includes bread, pasta, hot or cold cereal, corn, millet, barley, bulgur, buckwheat groats, and tortillas. Build each of your meals around a hearty grain dish—grains are rich in fiber and other complex carbohydrates as well as protein, B vitamins, and zinc.

Fruit. Fruits are rich in fiber, vitamin C and beta-carotene. Be sure to include at least one serving each day of fruits that are high in vitamin C—citrus fruits, melons, and strawberries are all good choices. Most of the time, choose whole fruit over fruit juices, which don't contain as much healthy fiber.

Vegetables. Vegetables are packed with nutrients; they provide vitamin C, beta-carotene, riboflavin, and other vitamins as well as iron, calcium, and fiber. Dark green leafy vegetables such as broccoli, collards, kale, mustard and turnip greens, chicory, or bok choy are especially good sources of these important nutrients. Dark yellow and orange vegetables such as carrots, winter squash, sweet potatoes, and pumpkin provide extra beta-carotene. Include generous portions of a variety of vegetables in your diet.

Legumes. Legumes, which is another name for beans, peas, and lentils, are all good sources of fiber, protein, iron, calcium, zinc, and B vitamins. This group

also includes chick-peas, baked and refried beans, soy milk, tofu, tempeh, tex-
turized vegetable protein, and peanuts. (Remember: Peanuts and peanut butter
are still high-fat sources.)

FOOD GROUP	NUMBER OF SERVINGS	SERVING SIZE
Whole grains	5 or more	½ cup hot cereal
		1 ounce dry cereal
		1 slice of bread
Fruits	3 or more	1 medium piece of fruit
		½ cup cooked fruit
		½ cup fruit juice
Vegetables	3 or more	1 cup raw vegetables
		½ cup cooked vegetables
Legumes	2 or 3	½ cup cooked beans
		4 ounces tofu or tempeh
		8 ounces soy milk

Round your diet out by including a good source of vitamin B_{12} (cobalamin). Most multivitamin/mineral supplements include this nutrient; enriched
soy or rice-based milk substitutes and many cereals are also fortified with B_{12}.

Sometimes having a simple list like the one above is helpful, especially if
you're feeling unsure of taking what seems like a major leap. Use these serving
numbers to help you plan healthy meals but don't get caught in a dietlike trap.
These are guidelines. Rest assured—natural foods are nutritious foods. If you
eat a variety of them, you will not ordinarily have to weigh, measure, or count
servings.

It is gratifying to see knowledgeable professionals formulate nutritional
guidelines that are ideal for both human and planetary health. Even without a
system of food groups, however, it is not difficult to plan an adequate diet from
natural vegetarian foods. Nature has designed these to meet our needs, not just
adequately but abundantly. Of course, some planning is required, particularly
because low-fat vegetarian foods are not yet the major menu items at fast-food

restaurants and roadside diners, which often seem the most convenient places to stop. Your choice of restaurants will gradually change as your style of eating changes, and you may find that you like your own cooking more and more.

In spite of abundant information to the contrary, many people fear that in making the transition to simpler eating, they will miss out on specific nutrients, like protein, iron, calcium, riboflavin, and vitamin B$_{12}$. Here's a look at each and how to ensure that you'll get enough.

PROTEIN AGAIN

WE'VE TALKED ABOUT GETTING TOO MUCH, so now let's talk about getting enough. If you could design a diet built around natural starches and vegetables that provided enough calories to maintain normal weight but was deficient in protein, you'd be famous because no one has been able to do so yet. The only way a person on a natural-foods, animal-free diet could become deficient in protein would be to take in too few calories due to excessive fasting or dieting or by living solely on those few fruits or other natural foods that are quite low in protein (less than 5 percent of calories).

But what about amino acids, those building blocks of protein that some people believe total vegetarians can only obtain by eating grains, legumes, and nuts in precise mathematical combinations? You can save your calculator for doing your taxes. You won't need it to prepare your dinner. Eat a variety of natural foods over the course of the day and protein complementing will take care of itself. "In fact," says Eisman, "all plant proteins are complete. Some are higher in certain amino acids than others, but by eating enough of any one plant protein, all needs can be adequately met. The irony is that an incomplete protein does exist: It's gelatin, an animal derivative." (For a helpful protein summary, see page 129.)

THE POPEYE PRINCIPLE

NATURAL VEGETARIAN FOODS MAKE A RESPECTABLE SHOWING in terms of iron content—dried fruits (prunes, raisins, apricots, and peaches), dried beans and lentils, whole grains like rye and wheat, and green leafy vegetables are all rich in this mineral. It has long been held, however, that iron from animal sources (heme iron) is more readily assimilated than nonheme iron from plants. Also, phytates (a form of phytic acid) present in whole grains have been believed to detrimentally inhibit iron utilization, although this has never been shown to cause iron deficiency in humans.

"In research, the focus is often on single or isolated nutrients or other substances," says Suzanne Havala, R.D., who has done research into the iron sufficiency of vegetarian diets, based in large part on the Chinese study. "Results often ignore the reality of the complex nutrient interactions that occur within the context of the total diet. In this case, plant components such as fiber and phytates apparently do not have a significant effect on iron absorption in vegetarian diets that contain adequate vitamin C from fruits and vegetables. Vegetarians in the United States tend to have good iron status."

Just as iron absorption can be impeded, it can also be enhanced. One way to do this is to eat one or more foods rich in vitamin C, such as citrus fruit, tomatoes, or green peppers, along with an iron-rich food. Another way to add iron to your diet is to use cast-iron cookware. "It was found that a 100-gram serving of spaghetti sauce prepared in iron cookware contained 87.5 milligrams of iron compared to only 3 when cooked in a glass vessel," reports Agatha Thrash, M.D., in her book *Nutrition for Vegetarians*.

CALCIUM OR COWCIUM?

PERHAPS EVEN MORE UBIQUITOUS than the myth that meat is necessary for protein is the myth that cow's milk is necessary for calcium. This defies logic in several ways. First of all, over half of the world's population, primarily those of African and Asian descent, lack the enzyme to digest cow's milk. Just because enzyme tablets or liquid can be taken to compensate for this does not make it a disease or abnormality. On the contrary, the ability to tolerate dairy foods may in fact be an adaptation to their consumption rather than an indication of normal digestive capacity. It is, after all, only the human species that drinks milk after weaning or takes the milk of another animal. All the calcium in cow's milk comes from the grass and grain eaten by the cow. Although you may not choose to refrain from eating dairy products, it is important for you to know that humans, as well as cows, can get all the calcium we need from plant foods.

In fact, virtually any vegetable food you might choose has some calcium in it. In his book *Vegan Nutrition: Pure and Simple*, Dr. Klaper lists these calcium all-stars: collards, kale, oats, chick-peas, trail mix made of one part almonds to two parts raisins, and calcium-fortified tofu. (Tofu made with calcium sulfate will say so on the label.) Calcium-fortified and enriched versions of soy milk and rice milk—tasty substitutes for cow's milk, available at health food stores and some supermarkets—are also easy ways to boost calcium intake.

Moreover, the total amount of calcium that you will need on a vegetarian diet is probably lower than you think. This is because the high-protein content of a meat-based diet causes calcium to be withdrawn from the bones. To eliminate the breakdown products of excess protein, the kidneys are forced to work overtime at excreting more urine. And minerals are in that urine, notably calcium.

In researching this, I was astonished to learn that the countries with the highest consumption of dairy products also have the highest rates of osteoporosis. This is not so amazing when you realize that those are also nations with high protein intakes. Animal protein may be more of a culprit in this regard than an equal amount of vegetable protein. In a study done at the University of Texas Southwestern Medical Center in Dallas in the 1980s, people who switched from a vegetarian diet to one containing eggs, red meat, poultry, and fish excreted more calcium, although the actual amount of protein ingested remained the same. (The high sulfur content of animal protein is thought to be the cause. In the body, sulfur turns into the acid sulfate, which must be buffered; calcium and other minerals are withdrawn from the bones to do this.)

Although the Daily Value for calcium is 1,000 milligrams, the World Health Organization recommends only 500 milligrams daily. A total vegetarian diet—unless you make a point of eating high-calcium foods every day—will probably provide less calcium than one containing dairy products, but it will also be free of excess protein and thus help to ensure a positive calcium balance within your body.

RIBOFLAVIN

Most Americans get riboflavin (vitamin B_2) in dairy products, meat (especially liver), and eggs, so some nutritionists have expressed concern that vegetarians will lack this vitamin. I think that this is on par with telling someone who is chauffeured to the office by limousine that she's "missing out" by not driving herself like most Americans. In fact, riboflavin is found abundantly in leafy greens, legumes, and nutritional yeast, and to a lesser but still significant extent in whole grains. Avoiding empty-calorie junk foods that displace nutritious foods in the diet is the best way to ensure adequate riboflavin intake.

VITAMIN B_{12}

Vitamin B_{12} is a fascinating nutrient about which more is probably unknown than known. But we do know the following facts.

- Vitamin B_{12} is an essential nutrient—without it, severe neurological damage can occur.
- Only a minuscule amount is needed—6 micrograms a day.
- In almost every case of reported B_{12} deficiency disease, the cause was not a dietary shortfall but the patient's lack of intrinsic factor, a substance produced in the body necessary for the absorption of this vitamin.
- Vitamin B_{12} is made by microorganisms and therefore is not known to occur naturally in foods of plant origin that have been scrubbed clean.
- It is stored in the body for long periods—three to eight years. After three years (or immediately in the case of children, pregnant women, and nursing mothers), total vegetarians need to include in their diets a supplementary source of vitamin B_{12}.

Beyond this, there are many unanswered questions. There have been many vegans who have not taken supplemental B_{12} and have fared well, almost without exception. (Probably the tiny amounts of B_{12} needed were supplied by the microbes living in the human mouth and intestinal tract.) Nevertheless, total vegetarians are advised to include a reliable source of biologically available vitamin B_{12} in their diets to meet the Daily Value. This usually means taking a tablet about once a week since the daily requirement is so small. B_{12} is apparently better absorbed when taken on its own rather than as part of a multivitamin/mineral supplement. The Daily Value can also be met with regular intake of foods fortified with this vitamin, including fortified soy or rice milk and many of the breakfast cereals at the supermarket.

ONE MORE THING

A FEW NEW VEGANS ACTUALLY HAVE TO LEARN HOW to get enough calories. You may be thinking, "I could use more problems like that," but if you do find that you're losing weight too rapidly—such as the rate of weight loss on a crash diet (more than one pound a week)—you may need to increase your portions. The same is true if you're losing weight and don't need to.

You will be eating more food on a low-fat, natural foods program than with any other approach you've taken to lose weight or maintain the weight that's right for you. The caloric equivalent of a 4-ounce hamburger and 12 measly fries is 2 cups brown rice, topped with 1 cup cabbage, 1 cup cauliflower, 1 cup mushrooms, and half an onion stir-fried with nearly a tablespoon of olive oil. Since oils are the most calorific foods anywhere, if you decided to steam the vegetables instead, you could double their amount or have a wheat roll on the side.

Of course you don't have to be concerned with juggling calories any longer. You'll eat, you'll finish, and then you'll follow your heart to some noble pursuit or great adventure. (Or maybe you'll just wash the dishes, but you won't have to think about food while you're doing it.) Should you need extra calories to maintain normal weight, increase your amounts of the more concentrated foods like bread and pasta, and (unless you have a medical contraindication to this) you can be more liberal in your use of the rich relatives—concentrated sweets like dates and dried fruits and oil-rich foods such as nuts, peanut butter, olives, and avocados.

VITAMIN YOU

Foods contain nutrients, but you, with your unique physical self and the mind that so influences your body, are a nutrient processor. You are nourished not by what is on your plate but by what you can assimilate into your body. Nutrient antagonists abound in most modern lives. Excess stress can create a need for more B-complex vitamins. Diuretics can deplete potassium supply. A sedentary lifestyle and the use of caffeine, alcohol, cigarettes, birth control pills, certain antibiotics, and even aspirin can drain vitamin and mineral reserves. So, it's obvious that your entire way of life affects your nutritional program.

Part of the beauty of loving yourself thin is that it is not primarily about what you eat. The changes in the foods you choose come about as a result of changes in your consciousness, in your awareness, and in your willingness to love yourself and others. When you no longer need to eat for a fix because of a quiet miracle happening to you mentally and spiritually, a Love-powered food style beautifully expresses your inner transformation in an outer sense. Ultimately, the most important nutritional element is vitamin YOU. It is activated by contact with a Higher Power, supportive friends, an appreciation of life and every creature that has it, along with supplementary doses of gratitude and wonder.

If you think whole grains, vegetables, legumes, and fruit sound too basic for fine dining, read the following buffet brunch menu from the news conference at which the Physicians Committee for Responsible Medicine introduced the New Four Food Groups. I'm not recommending seven-dessert spreads, and it's usually safest for food addicts to keep things simple. Nevertheless, low-fat, total vegetarian food can dress up quite elegantly.

- Creamy Banana Date Shake
- Chilled Melon Soup with Berries and Roasted Pine Nuts
- Assorted Vegetable Lasagna
- Tortellini in Pesto Sauce
- Ratatouille Ravioli with Shallot Confit

- Red Bell Pepper Sauce
- Stuffed Grape Leaves with Rice and Almonds
- Vegetarian Chili
- Potato, Leek, and Tofu Tart
- Orange Crème Brûlée
- Lemon Trifle, Lemon Zest, and Strawberries
- Piña Colada Mousse with Pineapple
- Fruit Kebabs with Toasted Coconut
- Apricot and Mango Sauce
- Carrot Cake with Maple Syrup
- Strawberry Shortcake

NUTSHELL NUTRITION: THE MACRONUTRIENTS

IF YOU'RE A FOOD ADDICT, you have probably read quite a bit about nutrition. (Even at age 10, I memorized nutrient charts while my friends read comic books.) You may, in fact, be quite fed up with the entire subject. If so, this minisection is for you: nutrition in a nutshell or, to keep things low-fat, nutrition in a pea-pod. We'll start with the big guys or macronutrients: carbohydrates, protein, and fats.

Carbohydrates

Unrefined carbohydrate foods are our foremost energy source and also the storehouses of other vital nutrients. Carbohydrates come as either sugar or starch. Sugars are simple and can be utilized by the body almost immediately. Starches are broken down into sugars during the digestive process. Natural sugars are deliciously packed in fruit, with the highest concentration found in dried fruit. Starch is found in grains, vegetables, and legumes.

Refinement is good for social climbing but bad for carbohydrate nutrition. White sugar is the ultimate in this kind of refinement, so cut down on soft drinks and conventional baked goods. Use sweeteners such as dates, fruit concentrates, maple syrup, and barley malt when you cook, but remember that all sweetness comes from sugar and even sweeteners from Mother Nature's kitchen can be overdone.

Also, read labels. Corn syrup, brown sugar, raw sugar, fructose, dextrose, sucrose, and lactose are all forms of sugar, so beware of any packaged food product with a concentration of one or more of these. (Ingredients are listed on the label in order of the amount contained in the product. Some manufacturers are clever, though, and may use two or three types of sugar so no single one has to be listed as the first or second ingredient.)

Highly processed grains, like white flour, white rice, and degerminated cornmeal, have also been robbed of nutrients. In "enriched" foods, some nutrients are replaced, but enrichment is like having the person who steals your car give you bus fare. Stick with the whole grains and simple cereals, but beware of granola—it's usually high in fat and terribly sweet. Also note that even refined carbohydrates are generally superior to fatty foods. You would be better off with vegetable chop suey over white rice than with sweet-and-sour pork, or with white-flour pasta and marinara sauce than with veal parmigiana.

Protein

The golden age of protein—when we believed that eating lots of it would dissolve body fat and having it in shampoo could glue split ends together—passed, but a revival seems to be brewing. The wise will eschew this particular trip down memory lane.

Protein is simply a nutrient that is necessary for, among other things, growth, tissue repair, and combating infection. The Daily Value in the United States is 50 grams—well above the World Health Organization's recommendation of 39 grams a day for males and 29 for females. But meeting either standard on a varied natural vegetarian diet isn't hard. It may actually be good to avoid going over the Daily Value very often since calcium depletion and kidney damage are among the problems that have been linked with excess protein consumption.

Amino acids are the units that make up protein. Eight of them, called the essential amino acids, must be supplied by the diet. It was formerly believed that only animal foods provided complete protein (or all the essential amino acids) and that the only way vegetable foods could be made sufficient was to combine different foods (generally grains and legumes) at the same meal to create an amino-acid profile that looked like that of meat. This is not necessary. Simply eat a variety of foods throughout the day and in your diet overall. Although there are many vegetarian foods that are concentrated proteins, such as peanuts, dried beans and peas, and soy products like tofu, these do not need to be emphasized. In fact, a cup of beans a day is plenty. And with a variety of whole, natural foods, you'll get ample protein even on the days you leave beans off the menu.

Fats

Fats provide warmth and a concentrated energy source as well as essential linoleic and linolenic fatty acids. Saturated fats, which aren't necessary for essential fatty acids, are found primarily in animal foods, like butter, cheese, and meat, and in a few plant products, primarily coconut, chocolate, and palm oil. Unsaturated fats are abundant in vegetable oil, margarine, nuts, seeds, and avocado. Although saturated fats have been linked with high cholesterol levels and increased risk of heart disease, all fats are suspect factors in certain cancers. The safest course to take is to keep total fat intake modest. The most efficient way to do this is to eliminate fried foods and animal products and to be frugal in the use of higher fat plant foods such as peanut butter and oil-based salad dressings. Using some olive oil in cooking is acceptable for most people, but measure it by the spoonful: It's a quality fat but it's still all fat, so don't overdo it.

Fiber

Fiber (or roughage) isn't really a nutrient, but this indigestible part of plants is important in digestion and elimination. A natural foods diet of vegetables, fruits, whole grains, and legumes is by definition a high-fiber diet, even without supplementary fibers such as wheat bran for bowel regularity or oat bran to lower cholesterol. (Besides, this is a zero-cholesterol diet, which, for most people, should eliminate the need for an extraneous cholesterol-lowering agent.) Meat and most other animal products are virtually fiber-free. Fiber is also lost in processing, so try to choose whole fruits instead of fruit juice and whole-grain bread instead of white, and leave the skins on your potatoes.

THE MICRONUTRIENTS

WHEN IT COMES TO VITAMINS AND MINERALS, SMALL IS MIGHTY. They don't take up much space in your body, but they're important. A natural foods diet is full of vitamins and minerals. And when you consider that nutrition is still a young science with more vital food components yet to be isolated, it's important to choose natural foods that haven't lost their best parts to the mill or the cannery.

Minerals

Minerals are body-building elements that also aid in digestion and temperature regulation. Among the major ones are:

Calcium. Bone and tooth formation, blood clotting, muscle contraction, and nerve transmission require calcium. Because high protein intake depletes the body's calcium stores, people with an adequate but modest protein intake (provided in a natural vegetarian diet) are believed to require less calcium than meat-eaters need. The Daily Value for calcium is 1,000 milligrams; the World Health Organization's recommendation, however, is only 500 milligrams per day. Foods rich in calcium include green leafy vegetables (collards and kale top the list), sea vegetables (kelp, dulse, nori), nuts such as almonds and filberts, legumes such as chick-peas and pinto beans, tofu cultured with calcium sulfate, calcium-fortified orange juice, and calcium-fortified soy and rice milk.

Iodine. A tiny but essential amount (100 to 300 micrograms) is needed for energy production and proper functioning of the thyroid gland. It's added to iodized salt but is also abundant in sea vegetables and in vegetables grown in coastal areas with significant levels of iodine in the soil. (*Note:* Most people get more than enough iodine in their diets and probably don't need to seek out these foods high in iodine.)

Iron. Needed by the blood for its oxygen supply, this mineral also aids in disease resistance and red blood cell formation. Iron is found in leafy greens (collards, kale, broccoli), legumes (chick-peas, lentils, lima beans), and other foods including whole grains and fruits—dried fruits in particular. Consuming food rich in vitamin C along with iron-rich food increases iron absorption by the body. The Recommended Dietary Allowance for iron is 10 milligrams a day for men and 15 milligrams a day for women.

Magnesium. Required for the body's acid-alkaline balance and for blood sugar metabolism, magnesium is part of the nutrient package of peanuts, almonds, legumes such as soybeans and lima beans, millet, wheat, and rye. The Daily Value is 400 milligrams.

Phosphorus. Though used in a variety of body processes including energy production, phosphorus is mainly calcium's right-hand mineral, important in bone and tooth development. Phosphorus is widely available in foods, and meeting the 1,000-milligram Daily Value for adults is not a problem. Rich sources include whole grains, legumes, peanuts, and peanut butter.

Potassium. Potassium is necessary for proper functioning of the heart and other muscles and for nerves. You can find it in sea vegetables, soybeans and lima beans, dried apricots, sunflower seeds, and prunes.

Selenium. A trace mineral with antioxidant properties, selenium is a component of whole grains, broccoli, nutritional yeast, and onions.

Sodium. Sodium is lost in sweat, urine, and feces and is replaced by foods, but most people get far too much. Table salt is the recognized source of sodium, but milk and its products, meats, canned vegetables, baked goods, and snack foods up the average intake considerably. Adequate sodium is provided by fresh vegetables. Use salt and soy sauce with a light hand.

Zinc. Needed for proper growth, reproduction, and wound healing, zinc is in oatmeal, peanuts, peas, dried beans, pumpkin seeds, and even popcorn. One study showed that phytates in whole grains inhibit zinc absorption, but this has not been evidenced clinically.

Vitamins

Vitamins are vital to normal metabolism. They are either fat-soluble (vitamins A, D, and E) or water-soluble (vitamins B and C); the latter are more easily lost through careless preparation. Prolonged soaking and boiling are vitamin murderers; try to steam, bake, and stir-fry when you can. It's a good idea to turn your leftover cooking water into soup stock. Better yet, eat raw vegetables whenever possible.

A good salad—leaf or romaine lettuce instead of pale iceberg—is a vitamin pill with dressing.

Vitamin A. For healthy skin, eyes, and respiratory tract, think yellow and dark green—as in sweet potatoes, carrots, cantaloupe, dried apricots, kale, collards, and spinach. The Daily Value for vitamin A is 5,000 international units (IU).

Vitamin B complex. Needed for digestion, protein breakdown, and nervous system functioning, the Bs aren't called complex for nothing. They're a conglomerate of vitamins. Nutritional yeast (a fortified and tastier form of brewer's yeast) is the classic vitamin B health food, but members of the B family also congregate in whole grains, wheat germ, and peanuts.

Following is a B-by-B breakdown, including some of the richest sources of each.

B_1 (thiamine) contributes to a good appetite and carbohydrate metabolism. Rich sources are brown rice, sunflower seeds, soybeans, and other legumes.

B_2 (riboflavin) contributes to antibody and red blood cell formation, cell respiration, and metabolism of all food elements. Good sources are almonds, whole-wheat bread, wild rice, leafy greens, and legumes.

B_4 (niacin) is needed for cell metabolism and respiration as well as carbohydrate absorption. The niacin deficiency disease, pellagra, was common prior to the enrichment of refined grains. Good sources are brown rice, wild rice, peanuts, millet, and collards.

B_6 (pyridoxine) contributes to antibody formation and hydrochloric acid production. Good sources are peppers, leafy greens, cauliflower, citrus fruits, and potatoes.

B_{12} (cobalamin) is required by the nervous system and by the blood in miniscule but essential amounts. Since it is produced by microorganisms, most people can probably get all they need from the microbes that live in their mouths and intestines. Because B_{12} does not reliably occur in vegetable foods, the wise course for a total vegetarian is to take a supplementary B_{12} tablet to meet the Daily Value of 6 micrograms or to regularly use foods fortified with cobalamin.

Vitamin C. Involved in collagen production, digestion, healing, and infection resistance, vitamin C gets to the table in citrus fruits, cantaloupe, strawberries, bell peppers, cabbage-family vegetables, and potatoes. The Daily Value for adults is 60 milligrams per day, although a substantial body of research indicates that a higher intake is optimal.

Vitamin D. The sunshine vitamin is essential for teeth and bones, so it is especially critical for children and pregnant women. Vitamin D is also needed for calcium metabolism and heart action. Although dairy products and margarine are fortified with it, nature intended for us to get our supply of vitamin D from the sun. Since most of us don't get sun year-round, vitamin D is stored in our tissues.

Vitamin E. Vitamin E is an antioxidant that regulates destructive oxidizing of cell membranes and vitamin A. It's widely available, particularly in whole grains, wheat germ, sweet potatoes, leafy greens, and navy beans. The Daily Value for adults is 30 international units.

EIGHT
Eating to Live

I AM GOING TO BE PRAGMATIC NOW AND DEAL WITH GROCERY CARTS, restaurant menus, and the culinary basics of loving yourself thin.

Eating destructively has been the problem, but eating constructively is an essential part of solving it. For this reason, we need to talk about food. If you are a food addict, be sure that you feel ready to read and think about food right now. As long as you are in the state of spiritual fitness that the book *Alcoholics Anonymous* refers to as "a position of neutrality, safe and protected," you can open yourself without fear to all the useful information you'll need. You're not fraternizing with the enemy by learning a better way of eating and cooking techniques—you're developing a new and healthier relationship with food.

We're going to be viewing food from a perspective that may be unlike any you've taken before. Knowing how a food tastes, how much fat is in it, and what vitamins and minerals it provides has its place. Recognizing how we feel about certain foods is equally important.

Take, as an example, string beans. If you're going to use the fresh ones, they need to have their ends removed. It's tedious but I'm convinced that such chores are far more meaningful than they appear because they speak of our connection with nature—a connection that is stabilizing and healing.

Of course it's easier to open a bag of frozen beans. They don't have any more calories than fresh ones, and nutritionally they're virtually identical.

135

Sometimes saving minutes is a legitimate priority, but the price paid for the convenience is that we give up the tactile and participatory experience of taking the fresh option. We tend to think that aerobic exercise is the only activity that helps keep a body fit and trim. That's not so. Snapping beans and shelling peas will do it, too, just in a different way. They put us in a sort of psychic kinship with the foods we eat, with the soil, the seasons, the source of physical life and nourishment. Binge eating is in direct opposition to this kinship, because it shuts us off from life.

A GENTLE TRANSITION

YOU WILL SOON EXPERIENCE A LOT OF CHANGES—changes in your outlook toward food as well as in your diet. Before we look at the dietary shift, let's work a little with change itself. To do this, it will help to make some lists.

First, jot down three really important positive changes that you've made in your life, actions that in retrospect you're glad you took. Now, think back to when each was just beginning. How was it? Did you love whatever it was without reservation or was there a period of adjustment? Was your positive change (going off to college, moving to another state or country, making a midlife career move) comfortable from the start or did you have to get used to it?

My list of important positive things includes (1) living in London after I graduated from high school, (2) becoming a parent, and (3) giving up my regular magazine job to freelance full-time. These are among the red-letter events of my life, turning points for which I'm deeply grateful. Nevertheless, when I arrived alone in the huge capital of a foreign country at the age of 18, I wanted to turn around and run back through customs in the other direction. When my daughter was born, I realized that not one of the dozens of books I'd read while pregnant had prepared me for the reality of caring for a tiny human being. And once I left the security of a steady job for the sink-or-swim uncertainty of self-employment, I felt that I'd joined a trapeze act that didn't use a net.

These separate and qualitatively different events took place over a 20-year time span, yet each required patience and persistence from me for its richness and beauty to become apparent. You probably noticed this during the important positive events in your own life. Now you're about to chalk up another as you commit yourself to turn from forcing yourself thin to loving yourself thin. The change for you in terms of diet could be relatively minor (maybe you're already a vegetarian but you're still attached to hefty quantities of cheese or ice cream) or it may call for a 90-degree turnaround in your eating habits. Whether subtle or startling in its particulars, this change will be significant. Allow yourself a gentle transition.

If choosing to eat in a way that expresses love to yourself and others is a commitment that grows from your deepest self, you'll realize that you're in this for the duration. You don't have to know everything right away. You don't have to be an expert. You only need to choose the very best foods you know of for today's three meals. Tomorrow, you'll know a little more and your choices then will reflect that.

I'd like to help you ease into this transition by reminding you of the Love-powered eating with which you're already familiar. There are times in your life, probably many such times, when you are not eating for a fix, when you eat some fresh, natural food and really enjoy it. That's how it will be nearly all the time when you're loving yourself thin. You already know how to do it. That's what you can build on. Let's start with exploring the New Four Food Groups—fruits, vegetables, whole grains, and legumes—in a gustatory way.

Fruit—Nature's Candy Store

Chances are, you eat fruit now and you probably like it. Nearly everybody does. It is possible to become so jaded by overindulgence in refined sweets (candy, pastries, and the like) that the delicate flavors of fruit are no longer appealing. After a few days away from sugary foods, though, fruit becomes a real treat. It's sweet and delicious, a veritable vitamin factory, and virtually fat-free. Fruit makes an ideal breakfast, a handy snack, or a light dessert that's always ready. You don't have to do anything to it, just enjoy.

Write down your 10 favorite fruits. That sounds like quite a few, but it won't be hard once you get started. Think of the exotic fruits you had on your trip to Hawaii. Remember that interesting melon you found at the green grocer's last summer, and the wild strawberries you picked at your grandmother's so long ago. You'll find that you already know some of nature's tastiest tidbits—and there are lots more where those came from. Now allow me to introduce you to my 10 favorites.

Bananas. Most people aren't aware that there are more than a dozen varieties of banana, each distinct. In northern climates, our selection isn't terrific (a banana is a banana), but even these make my list because when frozen, they turn a simple blender drink into something frothy and luscious. They can even become a treat that is astonishingly like ice cream. Use really ripe bananas (the skins need to be well-flecked with brown), peel them, and then freeze them in air-tight containers. If you have a clever appliance called the Champion Juicer (see "Good Food Gadgets" on page 178), you can run uncut frozen bananas through it (with the "homogenize blank" in place) to get delectable soft-serve. As an alternative, chop the bananas into 1" rounds before freezing, then puree them in your food processor, using the metal blade. You will need to scrape down the sides with a spatula every so often until the banana is processed into soft-serve consistency.

Cantaloupe. Cantaloupe probably wouldn't make my top 10 list if it weren't for the smooth and tasty shakes that can be made from the juicy, ripe ones. Chop a cantaloupe into cubes and put these in a blender with the smallest amount of water necessary to get the blender to liquefy the fruit. It's really amazing how thick and creamy this turns out—an exquisite light breakfast or summertime cooler.

Cherries. Cherries remind me of my dad, of visiting home and going with him to a certain produce merchant at the city market for the darkest, sweetest Bing cherries in season. Because of their pits, cherries can't be bolted down. It seems to me like nature's way of saying, "I put a lot into these, so slow down and relish them."

Dates. Dates are rich relatives (since they're higher in natural sugars than the basic foods) and lack the high water content of most fresh fruits. They're too rich to eat as snacks (except for active children, athletes, and people trying to gain weight), but four or five big Medjool dates with lettuce leaves, peanut butter–stuffed celery, and a crunchy Rome Beauty apple or two make my favorite light autumn lunch.

Mangoes. These are best when very ripe. You can often get them on sale when they look past their prime but are really just right for eating. Make a crosscut into the fruit starting on top and going one-quarter of the way down the sides. You can peel a mango by hand from there. Have plenty of napkins nearby. Mangoes are juicy, messy, and delectable. (A peeled, ripe frozen mango can be put through a good quality juicer for a heavenly sorbet.)

Papayas. Papaya is an acquired taste, and it's true that most of those shipped north can't compare with the tree-ripened tropical gems. Still, if you let one completely ripen until it is yellow and spotted and has the same give as a ready avocado, it can be a real delight. (Don't eat the black seeds that you'll scoop from the center; they're bitter.)

Persimmons. Life is too short to consider persimmons too expensive. I had never tasted this fruit until I was 30 and visited a resort in south Texas where custardlike persimmons were lunchtime specialties. I still get them often in late fall and winter, and although they do cost more than less exotic fruits, I think the persimmons and I are both worth it. (Eat them when they are very soft. When you think they're ripe, give them another couple of days.)

Raspberries. I love how these fragile, fragrant berries taste. I can remember getting a half-pint from a roadside stand in Indiana on a road trip once and savoring every berry right there by the side of the highway. That's when I realized that this slow savoring was the exact opposite of binge eating. I have Indiana raspberries to thank for the insight.

Strawberry fruit. This fruit gets its name because the flowers on its tree look like strawberry blossoms. This tropical treat doesn't ship well so you probably won't have ready access to it and neither do I, but when we both get a dream vacation to somewhere that's always warm and sunny, we can look for these grape-size white fruits that taste like caramels. Stuffed in half a papaya, they make a breakfast to write home about.

Watermelon. Watermelon is an air conditioner that you eat. I never liked it much until I learned the secret of watermelon connoisseurship: Eat it by itself, not with other foods. Its exquisite juiciness can't be appreciated in the company of other foods. (And people who have trouble digesting melon often find that eating it alone remedies that problem.) A terrific watermelon will be heavy—that's the sweet juice weighing in.

There are also, of course, apples, oranges, grapefruit, tangerines, starfruit, honeydew, pomegranates, pineapples, kumquats, pears (prickly and otherwise), peaches, nectarines, apricots, grapes, kiwifruit, figs, plums, blueberries, blackberries, and more. There are fruits for every climate and all times of year. You can see already that nature is not miserly—and we've only discussed one of the many tasty offerings from her pantry. Here are some tips.

Remember that fruit can be a quick breakfast, the perfect snack, or a de-*light*-ful dessert. (If eating fruit on top of other food doesn't agree with you, save your dessert for a couple of hours after the meal.)

Eat fruit when it's fully ripe. Much fruit is picked green for shipping and, with the exception of citrus and apples, often needs to ripen after you get it home. Bananas ripen best in a brown paper bag, and placing a banana in such a bag with unripe papayas, avocados, or pears hastens their ripening as well. An acrylic-resin or plastic bowl (like Lucite) is great for fruit ripening—and makes a pretty centerpiece.

Wash dirt, surface chemicals, and waxes from fruit (and vegetables) with a diluted detergent mixture, then rinse well. Or use a special cleaning product that's available for this purpose at health food stores. If produce is heavily waxed, you're better off peeling it.

Eat whole fruits most of the time instead of drinking juice. Juice is really a rich relative because its fiber has been removed and the natural sugars in juice can enter your bloodstream very quickly.

When you do drink juice, dilute it by half with water. (Sparkling water and fruit juice over ice make a refreshing soda.) Sip juice slowly, and prepare it fresh whenever possible. Citrus juicers, manual and electric, are inexpensive and easy to find in department and culinary stores.

Other than for the occasional special dish, eat fruit that is fresh and uncooked. Frozen unsweetened berries and mixed fruit may be used in smoothies (blended fruit drinks) or when fresh fruit is not available. Use canned fruit, even the juice-packed kind, only as a last resort. All canned foods have been heated.

Because they're very sweet, treat dates and dried fruits as rich relatives. If you wish to release weight, have these only in moderation (half a dozen or so dates, figs, or prunes or a handful of raisins a couple of times a week). Dried fruit is best soaked—reconstituted with water to more clearly resemble its fresh state—or save these rich foods for use in other dishes: Use them to sweeten hot cereal or garnish a salad, or add them to breads and muffins. If these sweets are binge foods for you, you're better off sticking with fresh fruits.

Plant a fruit tree. Plant 2. Plant 10. Some kind of fruit tree will grow almost anywhere. Start with a dwarf tree that will mature rapidly so you'll have something to pick without a long wait. Something momentous happens when you get fruit from a tree you've planted. You deserve that experience and the Earth needs every oxygen-producing tree it can get.

Everything's Coming Up Veggies

Many adults are still stuck in the six-year-old's notion that vegetables are "yucky." Vegetables carry the stigma in many people's minds of being "rabbit food"—dietetic stand-ins for something they would much rather eat. "I can eat 10 carrots when I'm on a diet," I was once told, "but when I'm not on a diet, I won't touch a carrot." Despite these tainted views, vegetables—leafy greens, in particular—are nutritional powerhouses, and according to the Center for Science in the Public Interest, the simple sweet potato tops the nutrition chart.

Let's face it: It takes some sophistication to truly appreciate vegetables. Children don't have it. The unimaginative who think of vegetables as canned peas and the lettuce on a burger don't have it either. But you do and we're going to explore that now. Think of a vegetable you honestly like. It needs to be one that you enjoy without cream sauce, gobs of butter, or deep-frying. What's the vegetable you enjoy raw or steamed until it's bright and crisp? Write it down.

My favorite vegetable is broccoli. When I used to fast, I didn't crave the chips and candy bars that had gotten me in trouble, but I dreamed of broccoli— lightly steamed with a squeeze of fresh lemon. Even then, my subconscious knew the good stuff. Nowadays, I fix broccoli at least twice a week and order broccoli with garlic sauce every time I go to a Chinese restaurant. My body seems to purr when it has had broccoli.

How often do you eat your favorite vegetable? Is it one that can be eaten both cooked and raw? Have you tried it both ways? Let's start a new list. Write down 10 other vegetables you like. Make two columns: one of 5 vegetables you like raw (or uncooked as I like to think of it), and one of 5 you like cooked. (Some could be listed in both columns, but be sure to put down 10 different vegetables altogether.) Here are mine.

FAVORITE HOME-COOKED VEGETABLES

1. Asparagus. Asparagus is a marvelous luxury. Try it slightly steamed with a touch of herbal seasoning like Vegit or Mrs. Dash.

2. Fresh peas. Eat them right from the pod, quickly steamed.

3. Chinese wood ear mushrooms. Chewy and hearty, wood ears have a consistency that helps some people get over a yearning for meat. I like them scored with crosscuts on top and sautéed in a little oil and sherry with a dash of lemon juice and a few snips of parsley. They can also be boiled for a minute and used in other vegetable or grain dishes, soups, or stir-fries.

4. Spaghetti squash. This big, oval yellow squash is lots of fun since its meat, when cooked, is like strings of spaghetti. Scoop the seeds from a halved squash, cut into quarters, and steam, or prick the skin and bake it whole. Serve with an herbal seasoning (plenty of garlic) or fresh tomato sauce.

5. Kale. Not only does kale pack in calcium, iron, and vitamin A, but it can be delicious, too. Dark leafy greens have the reputation of being strong and bitter (maybe that's why salad bars often have kale around the bowls for garnish instead of in them). Greens are misunderstood and underrated, though. Chop or shred kale (I use kitchen shears for this), steam in a vegetable steamer for 5 to 6 minutes, and season with a little lemon juice, ground black pepper, and salt (if desired).

FAVORITE RAW VEGETABLES

1. Arugula. This is no wimpy vegetable but a Mediterranean contribution to a super salad that makes its presence known. Its taste can vary—sometimes in summer becoming quite hot and spicy—giving a gourmet touch to any season's salad. Clean it well and use sparingly until you become an arugula aficionado.

2. Fresh corn, cut from the cob. When it's harvest time for corn and you can get it straight from someone's garden or just picked at a farmers' market, young corn is sweet and juicy and perks up a salad quite nicely. (Baking corn on the cob is another good idea. The result is a much more flavorful vegetable than when it's boiled. It also roasts beautifully over a fire or in coals on a picnic or camping trip.)

3. Sweet red pepper. Sweet red peppers usually cost a little more than their more prominent green brethren, but the taste—and additional nutrients—make up for it. They're also such a wonderful color. A salad of Christmas-green spinach, a few shreds of purple cabbage, and bright red rings of sweet pepper feeds your eyes before you even pick up a fork.

4. Cauliflower. This is my favorite of crudités. So unlike the overcooked, grayish mush that passed for cauliflower in the school cafeteria, raw cauliflower is tasty without being strident and has a dandy crunch.

5. Carrots. I go through a peeler at least once a year because our household carrot consumption rivals that of Peter Rabbit's. Usually, I eat a carrot whole, but I'm also apt to shred a couple in the food processor and use carrot instead of lettuce or sprouts on a sandwich; or I make carrot-raisin salad. (You don't need mayonnaise for this—just mix shredded carrots with raisins and toss with a little pineapple juice and, if you like, a handful of sunflower seeds.) I'm a fan of carrot juice as well. Like fruit juices, it's sweet and lacks fiber, but it's packed with beta-carotene and energizing enzymes. Carrot juice is also the tasty base for making blends with less-sweet vegetable juices. Carrot/beet and carrot/celery/parsley juices are wonderful. When I drink them, I feel as if I'm doing something really special for myself. Vegetable juices are best when made in a juicer and sipped slowly. A stemmed goblet doesn't hurt either.

Raw vegetables must be fresh in order to be palatable. I'll admit to cooking sagging spinach, yellowing broccoli, and limp carrots when they would never have been served for a salad or as crudités. You've probably done the same thing. There's nothing wrong with "waste not, want not," but it goes to show that vegetables that are delicious raw are the cream of the crop.

Now we each have lists of our 10 favorite vegetables to include in salads, on relish trays, as steamed side dishes, or in casseroles and stir-fries. Starchy vegetables like potatoes, yams, and winter squash have enough substance to be entrées on their own. Following a salad with a steamed vegetable platter served with rolls or rice is a lovely meal, particularly in late summer when garden vegetables are most abundant. A salad itself can be a main dish when a heavier food like pasta, brown rice, or chick-peas is included in it; and hot vegetable soup with your own cornbread or bran muffins makes a fine winter lunch or late supper.

If your thumb has the slightest hint of green, consider doing a little gardening. Use fresh vegetables as often as possible; get the freshest-looking ones you see. Stay away from canned vegetables: They are overcooked before they ever see your stove, and most are heavily salted. Experiment with vegetables. For every one you're not too fond of, there will be two or more that become your perennial favorites. Choose vegetables for their colors, textures, nuances of flavor, or even the way they feel. And don't forget the joy of snapping beans.

Grains Whole and Hearty

Grains are the foods that let you know that you ate. Whole grains are especially satisfying because they're substantial: You have to chew them. And when you chew grains, the digestive process starts right there in your mouth. The starches break down into their component sugars and the whole-wheat bread or brown rice you're eating tastes heavenly.

If you've always eaten refined grains like white rice and white-flour products, the natural grains may at first seem tough or coarsely textured. Don't feel that you have to change to eating all your grains as whole grains overnight. There will probably always be times at restaurants or in social situations when only refined grains are available. Unless the particular food is a binge provoker for you, it's okay. You're improving your diet, not engaging in an endurance trial.

Give yourself some credit. Maybe you already eat oatmeal every morning and you truly prefer whole-wheat bread, but you can't stand the thought of brown spaghetti. You're already ahead of the game. Give yourself some time. It won't be long before most of the refined stuff will taste like puffed air. Once you think of grains as generally referring to the whole grains that give an appetite what it came for and then send it on its way, it will be much easier for you to see grains as a main course.

Let's go back to the list. Write down three meals you like that have a grain entrée. You can include pasta, waffles or pancakes, a rice dish, fresh bread with soup, or even a special sandwich. Write it down even if the way you eat it now is high in fat or has animal ingredients. For example, you're probably used to pancakes made with milk and eggs. You can, however, make great pancakes that contain neither and use whole-wheat flour, too. Even pizza can be considered a grain-based entrée if it has a really good crust, is topped with sauce and vegetables, and has no cheese or just a little mozzarella.

There's probably a lot more variety in the grains available than you may think. In addition to the familiar ones like wheat, rice, oats, and corn, there are many unusual varieties, mostly found in stores that sell natural or gourmet foods. Experiment with an uncommon grain. Sometimes trying something new is a good exercise in risk-taking. Ruts have a way of making themselves deeper, and the same-old-food rut is one of the easiest to get out of. So make millet or kasha or quinoa for dinner. It will probably be a tremendous success. And what if it isn't? Peanut butter sandwiches were invented for just such situations. Keep the following grain facts in mind.

You don't have to skimp on your portions. You won't be eating gluttonously, but you'll be able to have ample, restaurant-size servings of pasta, enough rice to fill you up, and sandwiches that needn't be open-faced.

The old proscription against eating two starches at a meal no longer applies. You may not want both rice and potatoes or oatmeal and toast, but you can have them.

Promote grains from side dish to main course both in your thinking and in your meals. (Remember that starchy vegetables like potatoes, yams, and winter squash as well as the low-fat, high-carbohydrate chestnut all have entrée potential.)

Start the switch from refined to whole grains by revisualizing them. When someone says "bread," for example, consciously replace white with whole wheat in your mental image.

If you're afraid of grains (you think that they're fattening or you've often binged on bakery goods), be clear on the tremendous difference between solid, sustaining whole grains and empty carbohydrates like pale, lifeless breads and cakes and cookies that contain not only refined flour but refined sugar and plenty of fat as well. Unrefined grains are not apt to set off cravings, and they're only high in calories when accompanied by fats (as in fried rice or a muffin made with eggs and butter).

When you eat out, having a refined carbohydrate dish (white pasta or white rice, for example) is a reasonable compromise. You haven't blown anything. This is one way that your eating can alter slightly to fit your life, instead of altering your life to fit your eating.

The Love–Powered Bean Stalk

Like whole grains, legumes are substantial foods. It's not difficult to think of lentil soup or baked beans or chili as a main course. Beans do carry the stigma of being poor folks' food, but they're delicious just the same. And what's wrong with a bargain? Unfortunately, beans also have to live down their reputation for causing intestinal gas. It's true that they can be a culprit in this way, but there are things you can try to mitigate this, such as presoaking beans and then discarding the soaking water, eating beans in simple combinations (for instance, in a meal with only a salad and a nonstarchy vegetable), spicing them with the herb savory, sticking with sprouted beans (see "Sprout Farming" on page 163), or using more easily digested soy products like tofu instead of whole beans.

In fact, with versatile soy products such as tofu, soy milk, and meaty tempeh, you can make this major change for the better in your diet without bereaving the loss of many of the foods you're used to. Soy products—with the exception of some brands of fat-reduced tofu and low-fat and nonfat soy milk—are higher in fat than other legumes, but their ability to masquerade as a variety of animal foods makes these somewhat rich relatives well worth knowing.

If there are some foods you really think you'll miss when you eliminate animal products from your diet, write them down. Chances are, there is a reasonable facsimile (probably a soy product) sold commercially or one you can make yourself. I can't read your "miss list" but I can let you know that there are hot dogs, hamburgers, cheeses, milklike drinks, and even ice creams made from soy. And many vegetarian cookbooks have recipes for everything from kebabs and chicken salad to sauerbraten and gefilte tofu.

Other legumes can find a place on your menus, too. (For more on cooking with legumes, see "Bean Cuisine" on page 171.) For now, write on your sheet three bean dishes you like—even if you've never had them without meat. With plenty of herbs and spices, your pork and beans can be just as good without the pork. Split-pea soup is a tasty winter warmer that doesn't need ham, and great chili is a matter of beans, sauce, and seasonings, not ground beef. Just write down your favorite bean dishes to remind yourself that you would probably like to have them more often. (If you're curious about my list, it's Boston baked beans, taco salad with chili beans, and my mom's black beans and rice—all meatless and all really good.)

Remember the following facts about legumes.

• Dried beans and peas are solid and filling. They will help ease your transition from heavy foods and excess food to a lighter eating overall.

- Soybeans and most of the products made from them are higher in fat than other legumes. Look for fat-reduced tofu (⅓ less fat) and aseptic packs of 1% low-fat tofu.
- Legumes are a concentrated protein source. For this reason, don't overdo it. A cup of legumes a day is about right.
- If you haven't cooked beans much before, you may want to look into prepackaged bean soups and rice and bean combinations that come with their own seasoning packets.
- It's okay to use canned beans, but if you need to keep your sodium intake especially low, you will want to drain and rinse them.
- Most bean dishes at nonvegetarian restaurants have some kind of pork in them, and some Mexican restaurants still use lard in their refried beans. Ask before you order.

PUTTING IT TOGETHER

WHEN YOUR PANTRY IS FILLED WITH VEGETABLES, fruits, whole grains, and legumes, you'll be ready for delicious meals that will nourish your body and free your mind to pursue all the inedible—and, in fact, incredible— joys of life. Meal planning will not be a major issue.

I like to have a basic food plan that provides me with some structure (though not too rigid) so I don't have to think much about food. When it's warm, I usually have a fruit smoothie or shake for breakfast. Other times I make fresh orange juice when I get up and then later on have a more substantial meal like hot cereal with dried fruit, cold cereal with soy milk, a bran muffin, or toast with fruit preserves. On Sundays or holidays, I make pancakes or French toast.

When I'm really organized, I make a big salad right after breakfast so it's ready for lunch. I put in chick-peas or avocado and raisins so there's more to the salad than simply greens, and I eat it with a roll or crackers. Much of the time, I'm not that organized and don't think about lunch until I'm ready to eat it. Then I have leftovers from the previous night's dinner or I make a sandwich (a mixture of raw and sautéed vegetables in a tortilla is quick and delicious) or heat some soup. I usually make a big pot of soup on the weekend to have available throughout the week. Every now and then I'll have instant soup—there are some tasty ones at health food stores—with whole-grain rolls, raw vegetables, and bean or tofu dip. These foods travel well, too: You can put soup in a Thermos, salad in a plastic storage container, and sandwiches in waxed paper with the tomato packed separately to avoid soggy bread.

Dinner is almost always a large salad; an entrée based on whole grains, legumes, or potatoes; and a steamed vegetable. Sometimes there's dessert— apple crisp or nondairy ice cream—but not too often. You may be saying, "Rolls? Potatoes? Apple crisp? That's okay for you: You're not trying to lose weight. But what about me?" Let me assure you that this is precisely how I did lose weight. It was never dieting, though, because with the generous assistance of unconditional Love, my eating went from inappropriate to appropriate. I ate the food needed by a person with a normal-size body and my body became normal-size. I eat the same way today and I remain a normal size. Although you are likely to release weight quite easily after you begin to eat this way, it is not a quick weight-loss scheme. It is a way of life that is meant to be for life.

OUT TO EAT
• • • • • • • • • •

A FREQUENT OCCURRENCE FOR MOST PEOPLE these days is going out to eat. You can, too. Ethnic restaurants are the most fun because the cuisines of Italy, China, Thailand, India, Ethiopia, and the Middle East feature numerous totally vegetarian dishes. Moreover, you can eat well at almost any restaurant. Salad bars are healthy if you just avoid anything laden with mayonnaise or oil. Cafeterias and potato bars work, too. Steak houses always have baked potatoes and some kind of salad, as do most diners. Meatless burgers have found their way to most mid-scale restaurants' menus. Fast-food Mexican places can do bean burritos and veggie fajitas without cheese, and at least one of the popular burger chains will make a vegetarian rendition of their big sandwich—you can also order a salad at most of them.

At elite restaurants, the chef and other personnel will usually go out of their way to provide you with a vegetable plate or special pasta dish or salad even in those rare cases when there isn't one on the menu. Wherever you're eating, graciously ask for what you need and expect to get it. You can reserve a pure vegetarian meal when you make airline reservations. (Reconfirm this 24 hours before your flight.) You can also make an advance request for a vegetarian meal for almost any banquet or catered dinner.

I've had very acceptable meals in some very diverse situations. Once I attended a posh dinner reception after a movie premier to write about the event for a magazine. I had phoned the country club ahead of time to ask for vegetarian food. When the vegetable plate arrived (looking like the cover of a fine cookery magazine), my black-tied tablemates were obviously disappointed with their filet mignon. Several asked the waiter if there were any extra vegetable plates so they could make a trade.

In a completely different sociological environment, I was hungry in the midst of a journey by bus. My dinnertime layover was at a little depot and the only food available was provided by a hot dog vendor outside. He made me a hoagie sandwich of sorts: mustard, ketchup, relish, pickles, onions, and shredded lettuce piled on a frankfurter roll. It wasn't the Ritz, but it had a certain charm.

And some years ago on an extended car trip through the rural West, I was getting awfully tired of eating potatoes, toast, and less-than-fresh salads. I wandered into a truck stop in the wilds of Montana and right there on the menu in bold print was "Avocado and Sprout Sandwich on Dark Rye Bread." Given the setting, it was almost a surrealistic sandwich, albeit much appreciated. Whether you're eating in Love-powered fashion or not, you will have some enjoyable experiences in restaurants and some that aren't so great. A bonus of this way of life is that it won't matter very much. You will find that as your attitude becomes more and more empowered by Love, food may be more delicious than ever, but it will definitely be less important.

AMONG FRIENDS
• • • • • • • • • • • • • • •

WHEN YOU EAT WITH OTHER PEOPLE, those people and the conversation you share will be the highlights of the occasion, regardless of what is served. Food prepared for guests needs to be simple and inviting. By and large, people enjoy simple food. Even those who have no desire to revamp their own style of eating appreciate a natural, vegetarian meal as a change of pace. I think it also makes them feel that they've done something nice for their bodies, which indeed they have.

When you're invited to be a guest for a meal in someone else's home, know that you've been invited because you're liked, not because you'll clean your plate. Let your friend know that your dietary needs are different now, but make it clear that you don't need special treatment. Salads, breads, and grain and vegetable side dishes are usually more than ample at formal dinners. If the affair is informal, like a buffet or a potluck, select what you want and leave what you don't. Bringing a dish to share is not always appropriate, but most of the time it's a welcome gesture.

People are quite understanding today about others' dietary preferences. Give your friends and relatives the opportunity to be understanding of yours. When you adopt a Love-powered diet because you love yourself and every living thing, maintaining it is simply not difficult. I think it has something to do with commitment, a stand that in itself carries astonishing power. During a period of uncertainty in my life, my friend Sue shared a quote with me that I've really cherished: "When one truly commits oneself, then Providence moves, too." It has never failed: My commitment has to come first, then doors open that I never knew were there.

Your commitment isn't to stick to this diet no matter what. Your commitment is to be motivated by Love no matter what. You'll see the importance of this in your dealings with those closest to you. If you have a family or a close relationship with another person, you won't be alone when you alter the way you eat. Ideally, your spouse or parents or others with whom you live will read this book and come to realize why you're making the changes you are. Perhaps they will want to make some changes themselves.

Or they may see this as one more diet, one more phase. They might be threatened by changes they see in you, even those that they've asked you to make, such as losing weight. Your new way of eating could seem extreme to them, and they may let you know that they think you've gone too far. If this is the case, you can:

- Get the support you need elsewhere
- Eat the way you truly believe is best for you
- Remember to be grateful daily for the people you love, even when they aren't as supportive as you would like
- Refrain from the urge to try to convert anybody

In talking about the inner transformation you're undergoing, your life will speak for you. This is true of your new way of eating as well. Whether it's your trimmer body, your higher energy level, or your improved state of mind, the benefits will start to show. People will want what you have.

In the meantime, accept the people around you and be willing to put up with some inconvenience. If another family member usually does the cooking, share your needs with that person and make it clear that you don't want to make extra work for him or her. Be willing to cook some of your own food. Offer to take over kitchen duties a couple of nights a week: The regular cook will get a break, and you'll get to introduce this new way of eating to your family without pushing it.

If you wear the chef's hat most of the time and your family expects meat at dinner, serve it with love. For the last several years of her life, I cared for an elderly woman who had helped raise me. She didn't eat much meat but at times she got a hankering for bacon or sardines or stewed chicken. Although I was committed to Love-powered eating for myself, I fixed those things for her when she asked for them. When she was in the hospital at the age of 87, she told me she realized that being vegetarian was important to me, that preparing her meat had probably been hard, and how much she had appreciated it. Shortly after that, she passed away.

Some people could say that I would have shown more love to her by giving her healthy vegetarian food without exception. Maybe they're right. But at the time, I was following my heart. What she told me just before she died had a lot more to do with that intangible aspect of the human heart than with bacon or sardines.

When you are healthy and happy and free from obsession, you'll also be freer to love your family and friends and yourself. If you're not yet healthy and happy and obsession-free, love your family and friends and yourself anyway; it will help you get there.

Love the foods that nourish your body and the life that nourishment provides you. Love your fullness and your emptiness. Most of all, love God, by whatever name you choose, and see your emptiness filled and your fullness redeemed. When you love like this, you'll soon discover that you're no longer eating to fill a bottomless pit, to solve a hopeless problem, or squelch a nameless fear. You're eating to live.

CULINARY BASICS

YOUR PERSONAL COOKING STYLE can be part of your solution just as it was part of your problem. Food addicts who are good cooks let their disease take over that talent. They spend most of their time in the kitchen and specialize in preparing their binge foods. In recovery, however, people with a gift for food preparation can use it to put together beautiful works of art, creating healthful meals for themselves and for those they love. Since they're cooking because they want to and not because an obsession is forcing them to, the kitchen becomes one of many places for them to express creativity, artistry, and love.

On the other hand, there are food addicts who detest cooking. They stock up for binges at convenience stores and fast-food eateries, and in a pinch they can binge on anything in the kitchen that requires no preparation. When these people get well, they're not apt to become gourmet chefs. They can turn their lack of interest in cooking to an advantage, emphasizing simplicity in their meals.

To Market, To Market

You can put love in your diet and be well-nourished shopping only at your local supermarket. Hit the produce department first; you'll do most of your shopping there. Then make brief stops at frozen foods and other strategic points within the store. There will be entire sections you'll bypass, like the butcher's counter and the aisles of snack foods and soda. Grocery shopping will get much quicker and easier. You'll probably notice that your food bill will decrease markedly as well.

You may want to make quick stops at the store for small amounts of food rather than huge hauls every couple of weeks. I learned to shop this way when I lived in London nearly 30 years ago and my tiny flat didn't have a fridge, and I shopped this way as recently as last week. I bought baby greens for salad, fresh vegetable soup prepared by the market, Italian bread, raspberries and soy cream, a bottle of sparkling cider, and a bouquet of mixed flowers, to create a special mood. It made a lovely supper, with bread and soup left over for the next day's lunch.

Since you'll probably be eating more fresh produce than you have been, it's good to find out what days the produce gets to the store and stop in on those days. You can get by with shopping once a week: Use the more delicate produce like spring greens and asparagus first and the heartier vegetables like kale and carrots later. Shopping twice a week means you can eat what you want the day you want it. Besides, a whirlwind shopping trip and breezing out through the express checkout is a lot more pleasant than stocking up for the apocalypse.

Although it is not mandatory, you will find that your meals will be more interesting if you get to know the stock of a good health food store. This is where you're most likely to find vegetarian specialty items: soy milk, egg substitute to be used in baking, a wide variety of meatless burgers, and types of grains and beans that aren't available at most conventional grocery stores. You can also expect to find organically grown grains, beans, and produce.

Some of the prices at health food stores will seem high, but you will get value for your money and in many cases support small, careful companies whose profit margins are meager for the quality they offer. In some cases, you can actually save money at a health food store. In particular, when you buy grains, flour, and nuts from bulk bins, you can choose the exact quantity you want and avoid paying for expensive packaging.

A real money-saver for the energetic is a food co-op. There are storefront co-ops and private buying clubs that you can join. By working for the co-op a few hours a month, you can buy your food at a hefty savings. (Being part of a co-op is also a way to meet other people who are interested in living more naturally and healthfully.)

Supermarkets are getting smarter, and many offer an array of organic produce and bulk products. Get yourself an imaginary shopping cart and we'll make the weekly grocery run.

Don't feel that you would have to buy all of this on a real shopping trip; this is for practice. The sample list on the opposite page includes most of the items called for in common vegetarian recipes, and I've stuck with those foods that are most widely available throughout the United States. If there are other vegetables, fruits, whole grains, and legumes that you like, add them to the list. And if there are items listed that you don't like—or that are binge foods for you—make a different selection.

PRODUCE

- Apples
- Bananas
- Broccoli and other greens (kale, collards, Swiss chard)
- Cabbage, red or green
- Carrots
- Celery
- Lettuce (preferably leaf or romaine; iceberg is less nutritious)
- Mushrooms
- Onions (scallions, too, if you like them)
- Oranges
- Other seasonal fruits
- Peppers, green or sweet red or yellow.
- Potatoes for baking
- Specialty greens (arugula, cilantro, radicchio)
- Spinach
- Tomatoes
- Yams

FROZEN FOODS

- Frozen lemon juice
- Fruit juice concentrate
- Unsweetened frozen fruit
- Vegetables of your choice (plain, not with fancy sauces)

CANNED GOODS

- Beans (such as pintos, chick-peas, chili beans in sauce, and vegetarian baked beans)
- Soups (optional—most canned soups are quite salty; choose vegetable, lentil, and minestrone soups without chicken or beef broth)

• Tomatoes
• Tomato sauce and paste

PACKAGED FOODS

• All-fruit jam or preserves (these contain no added sugar)
• Aluminum-free baking powder (Rumford's is one brand)
• Apple cider vinegar or seasoned rice vinegar (this is a super salad dressing on its own), mustard, natural soy sauce (look for reduced sodium tamari)
• Brown rice (get the regular and quick-cooking kind), rice pilaf, and flavorful white rices like jasmine and basmati
• Dried beans and peas (lentils, split peas, navy beans, or your choice)
• Dry cereal (look for whole grains and a low sugar content; avoid granola unless it's specified low-fat)
• Herbal teas, Postum or Pero grain coffee substitutes, and bottled waters
• Herbs and spices of your choice (Mrs. Dash is a good salt-free seasoning; the most popular spices used in vegetarian cooking are garlic, ground black pepper, onion powder, basil, oregano, cumin, chili powder, curry, parsley flakes, and paprika—sweet Hungarian paprika is best)
• Natural peanut butter, English walnuts, and slivered almonds
• Oatmeal (quick or old-fashioned)
• Olive oil (look for cold-pressed oil; use the extra virgin oil in salad dressings, and use all oils sparingly)
• Pasta (use some that's whole grain)
• Raisins or other dried fruit, if desired (without the sulfur dioxide, which is sometimes used as a preservative)
• Real maple syrup or honey
• Rice cakes, whole-grain crackers, and popcorn to pop in your air-popper
• Whole-wheat bread (read the label: "wheat flour," "flour," and "enriched flour" all mean white; look for 100 percent whole wheat)
• Whole-wheat flour (if you bake yeast bread, using part unbleached white flour may be a good transitional step)
• Whole-wheat pastry flour (for quick breads and muffins)

REFRIGERATED FOODS

- Tofu (a refrigerated food but likely to be found in the produce section; also look for 1% low-fat tofu—Mori-Nu is a common brand name—in aseptic packaging)
- Whole-wheat and/or corn tortillas (sometimes frozen)
- Yeast, if you bake (note that baking yeast and nutritional or brewer's yeast are entirely different and not interchangeable)

NATURAL FOODS GLOSSARY

THE FRUITS AND VEGETABLES with which you're already familiar are true natural foods, and a healthful diet doesn't demand a boundless repertoire of different grains and legumes.

Nevertheless, becoming acquainted with some of the more unusual foods can give your meals a welcome variety. Some of these, take tofu for example, can also be used to create dishes reminiscent of those you'll no longer eat and may miss. You don't have to eat any of these things (many of them are, in fact, rich relatives), but they are available at your local health food stores for you to try.

Agar. A vegetarian gelatin made from seaweed. Agar, also called agar-agar, comes in sticks or flakes (the flakes yield the most consistent results). Use it like ordinary gelatin; one tablespoon of flakes will gel one cup of liquid.

Barley malt. A liquid sweetener made from sprouted barley, similar in flavor to molasses. Rice syrup is another natural sweetener and quite delicate.

Buckwheat. A hearty, quick-cooking grain with an earthy flavor. Also known as kasha, buckwheat can be cooked whole as a breakfast cereal or as a substitute for rice. As a flour, it's most popular in pancakes.

Carob. A chocolate-like treat from the pods of the locust tree. It comes in powder form for baking or making cocoalike drinks and is also made into candy. (The candy can be high in oil, however, and some contains sugar or milk.)

Egg substitute. Powder to be substituted for eggs in baking. Use one teaspoon egg substitute whisked with two tablespoons water for each egg. (Ener-G and Jolly Joan are two brand names.)

Granular sweeteners. Date sugar is ground dehydrated dates. It has a full-flavored taste, something like dark brown sugar. Fructose, generally derived from corn in spite of its name, looks and tastes like white sugar but is metabolized more slowly. Sucanat is made from sugar-cane juice that has been dehydrated and milled into a powder. It is richly flavored and very good in quick breads and bran muffins.

Millet. Little, round golden grains that cook up light and fluffy. Use as you would use rice at dinnertime, as a hot breakfast cereal, or as a base for other dishes such as vegetarian loaves and burgers. (And throw millet instead of rice at newlyweds since it won't harm the birds that eat it.)

Miso. Salty, fermented paste made from cooked, aged soybeans and sometimes from grains. Thick and spreadable, it's used for flavoring a wide variety of dishes and for making soup bases.

Nut butters. Bread spreads made from almonds, cashews, sunflower seeds, and peanuts. These are definitely rich relatives and very high in fat, but they can be used in moderation and in the preparation of other dishes. One that you'll see called for in recipes fairly often is tahini, made from sesame seeds.

Nutritional yeast. Imparts a sharp, cheesy flavor to sauces, soups, and casseroles. It can also be sprinkled on toast, popcorn, or spaghetti. Yeast flakes taste much better than the powder. Either form is rich in B-complex vitamins, and many brands are fortified with vitamin B_{12}.

Quinoa. Round, sand-colored grain with a mild, nutty taste and fascinating history going back to the ancient Incan culture. This cooks quickly.

Ramen noodles. Dry, wavy noodles that need only be boiled or steamed for a few minutes to reconstitute their texture and be ready to eat. They come in packages with seasonings included for a nearly instant meal.

Raw cashews. Nuts, or, more technically, the fruit of the cashew tree. Raw cashews are white and quite unlike roasted, salted cashews. High in fat, these are rich relatives like all nuts, but they're extremely versatile and relatively small amounts of them can be used to make "milk," white sauce, and a variety of other dishes. Buy the pieces rather than whole cashews to save money.

Rice milk. Milklike beverage made from rice. It's light and slightly sweet. Fortified rice milk is available with added calcium.

Seitan. Chewy, high-protein food made from baked or boiled wheat gluten. Seitan tastes much like meat when used in stews and casseroles or barbecued on a bun.

Soy milk. Milklike beverage made from soybeans. The label will usually state "soy beverage" (not milk). The fat content varies; look for the light varieties. Enriched soy milk contains added calcium, B_{12}, and other nutrients.

Tamari. Natural soy sauce, fragrant, flavorful, and far superior to typical grocery store soy sauce. Traditional tamari is wheat-free. Soy sauce made from soy and wheat is called shoyu. These seasonings are very salty, but reduced-sodium tamari is less so.

Tempeh. A fermented soy product with Indonesian heritage. Tempeh is very meaty in texture, barbecues beautifully, and is a natural for chili. But like most soy foods, it's fairly high in fat.

Tofu. Soybean curd that has made its way from Chinese restaurant menus to most supermarkets. This white cake is virtually flavorless on its own so it takes on the character of the condiments used with it. It can serve as the "meat" in a stir-fry, the "sour cream" in stroganoff, or the "cream cheese" in cheesecake. Look for reduced-fat versions. (See "Tofu 101" on page 172.)

Wheat-free breads and pastas. Breads, noodles, and spaghetti made from rice, rye, corn, and other grains. Wheat is a common allergen and many people are sensitive to wheat gluten. Health food stores stock breads, crackers, and pastas that contain no wheat.

GOING ORGANIC

ONE WAY TO SHOW SOME EXTRA LOVE to yourself, other people, wildlife, and the Earth is to purchase some organically grown foods. If you have some resistance to this idea, don't worry: I held out on it for a long time. It seemed to me that only health fanatics, leftover hippies, and the people my grandmother used to say had "more money than sense" would pay the usually high price for organic groceries. I figured that I was doing all right with regular food.

That was before I realized that synthetic insecticides, herbicides, and fertilizers weren't "regular" until some 50 years ago. Chemical-treated agriculture is a relatively recent phenomenon that grew after World War II. (The pesticide parathion, for example, was developed by the Nazis as a lethal nerve gas. It's 60 times more toxic than DDT, but still applied around the world to grains, produce, and cotton.)

And although the use of insecticides in agriculture has increased 12 times over during the past 30 years, damage to crops from pests has doubled during this time. Research from France now suggests that some ammonia fertilizers and certain pesticides may prevent plants from absorbing micronutrients. "This not only makes them less nutritious," says agricultural economist Terry Gips, president of the International Alliance for Sustainable Agriculture, "but it weakens the plant much like an immune deficiency, so insects can come to affect the weaker plants. It's a catch-22: The more you use, the more you have to use."

But consumers can opt for the organic alternative. Gips offers the following reasons for making the switch.

Personal health. Conventionally grown food contains residues of various pesticides. A Natural Resources Defense Council study found that 44 percent of California's fresh produce contained residues of 19 of these, including dieldrin and DDT, proven carcinogens.

Social justice. Nursing mothers in Central America have DDT in their breast milk at levels 42 times the World Health Organization's standards as a result of aerial spraying and residues in foods. In the United States, the National Cancer Institute found that farmers in Nebraska and Kansas who were exposed to the herbicide 2, 4-D run a 6 times greater risk of developing a rare form of cancer called non-Hodgkins lymphoma.

Wildlife protection. Runoff from agricultural chemicals concentrates in ponds, contaminating the food and water of migrating waterfowl and resulting in deformities.

Ecology. Farming with sustainable organic methods has many ecological advantages. Organic methods don't contaminate the ground or surface water, and they save energy since synthetic pesticides and fertilizers are made from petrochemicals (petroleum). Synthetic fertilizers also cause nitrates, which break down into carcinogenic nitrosamines, to enter groundwater. (A U.S. Environmental Protection Agency study showed that more than 50 percent of wells tested contain nitrates.) Organic methods also cause far less soil erosion, and organic farmers rotate their crops, which produces richer soil. Natural nitrogen fertilizers also make soil stronger, unlike artificial nitrogen, which breaks down humus, making it susceptible to loss from wind and rain. "Five bushels of topsoil are lost for each bushel of corn conventionally grown," says Gips.

Economics. Economics of scale in transportation and marketing means that the more people buy organic foods, the less those foods will cost. And demand creates supply: Every additional customer helps create the demand that will encourage more farmers to join the 50,000 in the United States who already farm organically. Health food stores carry organically grown grains, nuts, legumes, and often fresh fruits and vegetables. Food co-ops make these available at a lower cost. Organic produce and some other foods are available at select supermarkets, as well. Look for foods labeled "certified organic." The word natural has no legal definition. It's usually applied to products with no synthetic colorings, flavorings, preservatives, or other artificial additives. That's good, but it says nothing about the way in which the food was grown. "Certified organic" means that an independent monitoring agency has inspected a farm and determined that no synthetic fertilizers or pesticides have been used there in the past three years and that the farmer practices good soil management.

Now I can't tell you that you'll lose more weight or eat less obsessively when you fill your market basket organically. I do happen to believe that organically grown foods taste better. Maybe that's just because I like the way I feel about myself when I eat them. Or maybe some of the special care and attention that the farmers give the soil comes through in the rice and the carrots and the apples.

I also find that choosing organic foods puts me in closer touch with nature, with the land, and with my part in all that is natural. Feeling connected in this way brings with it a balance that is antithetical to obsessing over anything. If paying an extra 40 cents a pound for tomatoes can give me that, I'm getting quite a bargain.

THE ART OF THE SALAD

SALAD DOESN'T HAVE TO BE TOKEN GREENERY, bland, and perfunctory. In fact, it doesn't even have to be what we think of as salad. You can serve light and nutritious raw vegetables as:

Crudités. Carrots, celery, peppers, zucchini, broccoli, cauliflower, jícama (a starchy root), cucumbers, kohlrabi, mushrooms, and thinly sliced turnips are great alone or with dip. (With a beginner's book on garnishing and a few simple tools, you can make edible artworks from raw veggies.)

Sandwich fillers. Stuff some vegetables into a pita, roll them in a tortilla, or just put them between slices of bread. (Salad sandwiches are standard fare in Britain, especially ones made with cucumbers or watercress.)

One-dish meals. Make them main course by adding cooked beans (try garbanzos or spiced chili beans), brown rice, steamed new potatoes, curly pasta or elbow macaroni, or tofu cubes (marinate them in three parts water to two parts natural tamari soy sauce). Include bread or rolls on the side if you wish.

There's an art to the traditional tossed salad as well. You can experiment on your own or use recipes, but here are general guidelines for a salad you'll actually want to eat.

Choose vegetables that are in season. Or pick imported produce that looks fresh and appetizing. Also pick colors, textures, and flavors that complement each other. Visualize a salad made from iceberg lettuce, peeled cucumbers, cauliflower, and mushrooms. Pretty awful, right? There's no color there, no appeal. Now picture a salad with bright red tomato wedges, a cucumber crinkle-cut with its green edge intact, cauliflower set off by grated carrots and a few ripe olives, and mushrooms tossed into a bowl of spinach as green as a St. Patrick's Day hat. Now that's better.

Wash the vegetables you've chosen. Pay close attention to leafy ones like spinach and arugula that collect sediment in their crevices. Dry them before putting them in your salad bowl. If you use a wooden salad bowl, rub its interior with a cut garlic clove. It will impart a wonderful flavor to your salad.

Go easy on the oil. The main purpose of using oil in salad is to help herbs and seasonings cling to the vegetables. A tablespoon in a very large salad is sufficient for that. Try spraying on oil from a pump bottle instead of pouring it on.

You can actually do without oil altogether if you toss your greens with lemon or lime juice, sprinkle amply with salt-free seasonings, and a seasoned salt like Spike (if desired). Seasoned rice vinegar is a superb dressing on its own. Using cut tomato slices also provides liquid for this no-dressing dressing.

Avocado is another useful addition. A rich relative, it is high in oil content but it comes packed with the vitamins, minerals, and fiber of a natural food—something bottled oils can't claim. Even used moderately, avocado can give more satiety value to a salad than an oily dressing can.

You can also dress up a salad with tasty garnishes such as steamed vegetables (asparagus, string beans, broccoli) and small quantities of tasty rich relatives like sunflower seeds and olives. (Try topping a salad with whatever else is on the menu, like vegetarian chili or baked beans.)

Make it easy to eat salad. Keep washed vegetables in your refrigerator at all times. Salad tastes best when you eat it right after you put it together, but if you need to, make your lunch salad after breakfast and keep it in an airtight bowl until noontime. (If using dressing, add it right before you eat.)

Treat yourself to fresh fruit salads. Keep them simple: a melon salad of cubed cantaloupe, honeydew, and casaba melon; a tropical salad of pineapple, tangerine slices, and bananas; or an autumn salad of apples, grapes, and pears. If you use apples or bananas, add a squeeze of lemon to keep their colors true. Make a meal of a fruit salad with the addition of a cashew cream (⅛ cup raw cashew pieces to 4 ounces fresh orange juice, blended until smooth) and a sprinkling of sunflower seeds, raisins, or chopped dates.

SPROUT FARMING

YOU DON'T NEED A BACK FORTY or even a backyard to grow organic produce of your own. That is because sprout farming can be done anywhere. Even if you skip the alfalfa sprouts on salad bars and can take or leave the mung bean sprouts in Chinese food, you're apt to become much fonder of these "baby vegetables" if you grow them yourself.

Sprouts are seeds that have just begun to germinate, and these tiny plants are bursting with enzymes, vitamins, and minerals while shy on calories. Start with good organic seeds (get edible seeds and beans from a health food store, not chemically treated seeds meant for gardening) and count on getting a bundle—at least 5 pounds—of sprouts from every pound of seeds. Among the sprouts you can easily grow are:

Alfalfa. Use raw in salads. These sprout in two to five days.

Dried whole peas. Surprisingly sweet and crunchy, these need two to three days to grow to be ready for salads, snacking, or steaming.

Lentils. They take two to three days to sprout and are good raw or cooked; use them in soups and stir-fries.

Peanuts. My all-time favorite, peanut sprouts, like other sprouts, are low in fat since the sprouting process requires energy and gets it from the oil present in the unsprouted seed. These are ready in two days, no more than three. (Only raw peanuts will sprout.)

Radishes. Spicy. These will perk up an uneventful salad any day. Give them three to five days growing time.

Sunflower seeds. These sprout almost as deliciously as peanuts. They are leafy and crunchy at the same time and excellent in salads or on sandwiches.

You can also grow mung bean sprouts in two to four days, but since you may find it tedious to remove the bitter hulls, you may prefer to purchase these already sprouted.

Wheat and other whole grains sprout, too. They can be cooked when barely germinated (after the night's soaking and one day's sprouting time) or used raw as a strangely sweet sprout when allowed to grow for four to five days.

Soybeans are nearly impossible to sprout at home, but the soy sprouts that you can buy at Asian markets are tasty and substantial. These cannot be eaten raw; stir-fry them.

To grow a sprout garden, all you'll need are a Mason jar (a used peanut butter jar will do, unless you want a lot of sprouts, then use something the size of the large institutional food jars you can get from a restaurant or school), a piece of cheesecloth, and a rubber band. Then follow these steps.

1. Soak the seeds (one type at a time unless sprouting times are similar) in the jar overnight, or for at least 6 hours. It is important to use distilled or spring water for this purpose since chlorinated water can impair sprouting.

2. Cover with a piece of cheesecloth and attach with a rubber band. Drain the seeds and rinse them with fresh water (tap water should be okay for the rinsing). You'll want the seeds damp, not wet.

3. Turn the jar on its side at the edge of a sink or in a dish drainer. Rinse and drain two or three times a day until you're ready to harvest. (It's also a good idea to grow your sprouts in the dark—in a cupboard or beneath a dish towel—until the last day when you'll place them in a sunny window to develop chlorophyll and nice green leaves.)

As you may imagine, children love to grow sprouts. Sometimes, they'll even eat them.

A STEAMY ROMANCE WITH VEGETABLES

STEAMED VEGETABLES TASTE GREAT and take no talent on the cook's part. Steaming is also the most nutrient-saving cooking method. The only equipment needed is a stainless-steel steaming trivet available in any cookware department for just a few dollars. Simply place washed vegetables, whole or cut, in the basket over boiling water. The water shouldn't touch the vegetables. Cover tightly and steam until they're bright and crisp-tender. When preparing vegetables that require longer cooking, check the water level and add more water if it boils away. Here are steaming times for some popular vegetables.

Vegetable Steaming Times

VEGETABLE	STEAMING TIME (MIN.)
Beets, (medium, whole)	30–40
Beets (sliced)	5–6
Broccoli	10–15
Brussels sprouts	10–15
Butternut squash	20–30
Cabbage	10–20
Carrots (sliced)	10–15
Carrots (whole)	20–30

(continued)

Collard greens	8–12
Green peas, pea pods	5–10
Kale	5–10
String beans	12–15
Sweet potatoes (small to medium, whole)	25–30
White potatoes (small to medium, whole)	25–30
Zucchini	1–15

Stir-frying is another cooking method that is quick, easy, and produces a nutritious result. Unlike deep-frying, this technique does not require a large amount of oil. Less than a tablespoon should be enough in a heavy skillet, no-stick pan, or wok. Spread the oil over the surface of the pan and cook quickly, adding other liquids—water, sherry (or apple juice), tomato juice, or sodium-reduced tamari—and stir constantly. If you add extra water and cover intermittently, you're steam-frying, which is a good way to get maximum flavor with minimum fat.

SOUP STOCK

AN ORGANIZATION THAT WANTED a vegetarian luncheon for a seminar was told by a hotel chef, "You cannot make soup without chicken broth." They changed hotels and got terrific soup—without the chicken broth. You can make terrific soup, too. Frankly, a perfectly adequate one can be made just starting with water as a base and using miso or tamari for seasoning or a powdered vegetable broth mix or bouillon. These are available at health food stores. Brands include Vogue Vegebase and Jensen's Broth and Seasoning. Some of the powdered stocks taste like chicken or beef if you're looking for that familiar flavor.

If you want to take the homemade route, you can make a stock as good as your grandmother's by following this recipe: Save vegetable scraps and the water left from steaming vegetables. With the exception of cabbage-family members, such as broccoli and cauliflower, any vegetables will do. Clean potato peelings are really good, and so are the ends of beans and the tips of carrots. You can use onions, garlic, and mushrooms, too. Add your scraps (and any other vegetables you are using) to boiling water—about 2 cups vegetables to

4 cups water—and up to ½ teaspoon salt. Cover the pot and let the stock simmer just below the boiling point for about an hour. Let it cool, then strain and discard the vegetables.

Your stock will last in the refrigerator for one week, or you can freeze it in ice-cube trays. Use it as a base for all kinds of soups: corn chowder, garden vegetable, lentil, minestrone, navy bean, split pea, or potato. You can make cream soups by using soy milk, tahini, or blended raw cashews or by blending portions of a noncream soup (fresh pea or vegetable), adding a thickener such as arrowroot or cornstarch, and then reheating. Soups are one of the best reasons for having winter; and cold soups, like gazpacho and fruit soups, are perfect when it's hot.

THE PERFECT POTATO (AND TOPPERS)

To BAKE THE PERFECT POTATO (or a darn good one at least), choose firm russet or yellow Finn potatoes and cut out any "eyes." Prick the skins several times with a fork and bake in a baking dish (this seems to be the secret) in an oven preheated to 450°F. Baking will take about an hour, depending upon the size of the potatoes. If you plan to stuff them with other vegetables, they should be fairly large. You can lightly oil the skins if you want to, but don't wrap your potatoes in aluminum foil. There is some evidence that cooking in foil and with aluminum cookware can cause aluminum to build up in the body.

The perfect potato deserves the proper topper. Butter is an animal product and, for all intents and purposes, straight, saturated fat. Regular margarine, although made from polyunsaturated oils, has the same fat content as butter—100 percent. Diet margarine, although hydrogenated, has half the fat of ordinary margarine or butter. To make any margarine, however, oil is partially hydrogenated to make it solid at room temperature. Hydrogenation creates trans-fatty acids, which behave in the body like cholesterol-elevating saturated fat. When I want something that smells and tastes like butter, I use Spectrum Spread, a tasty soft margarine that is not hydrogenated. Or I go with one of the following unorthodox but tasty toppings.

- Salsa: Homemade or from a jar
- Broccoli: Oversteamed so you can mash it (broccoli stems left after you've cooked the flowerets work just fine) with plenty of ground black pepper
- Cauliflower: Just like broccoli
- Mashed sweet potatoes or yams: No kidding; cold leftovers work just fine—sort of like cold butter on a hot potato
- Tofu spreads: Experiment with the tofu mayonnaise (with plenty of chives) on page 174
- Pasta sauce: With plenty of garlic and basil
- Barbecue sauce: Those at health food stores have no refined sugar
- Steak sauce: At restaurants, steak sauce or mustard is sometimes the best you can do, but they're really not bad
- Ratatouille: Sautéed vegetables with tomato sauce, my favorite tater topper
- Avocados: "Green butter," mashed or thinly sliced or seasoned as guacamole

Use other seasonings, like Mrs. Dash, Spike, powdered vegetable broth, scallions, or chives, with these toppings and find your own specialties. A potato is fairly dry and mild-tasting, so you're looking for something to provide a little moistness and a touch of spice. Use your imagination.

SANDWICH IDEAS

EVERY ONCE IN A WHILE, YOU'LL STILL SEE on a menu the archaic diet plate of cottage cheese, a canned peach half, and a burger without a bun. It would be better to have a bun without a burger. A decent sandwich can, however, be well-filled and come with the bun or both pieces of bread. There are, in fact, a variety of breads from which to choose.

- Whole-wheat or whole-rye bread, or a gluten-free specialty bread if you're sensitive to wheat

- Whole-grain pita pocket
- Whole-wheat English muffin
- Whole-wheat burger bun
- Whole-wheat bagel
- Whole-wheat kaiser roll
- Whole-wheat or corn tortillas
- Other unleavened breads—matzo, chapati, or Ethiopian injera (a flat, spongy bread used as an edible utensil)
- Large crackers—rice cakes, Scottish oatcakes, or Norwegian rye crisp-bread (sold in large rounds)

Once you've found the bread, you need to fill, top, or spread it. There are dozens of ways to do this. You'll recognize several of the following as rich relatives, so don't overdo the quantities of high-fat or very sweet sandwich fillers. With a good bread and plenty of lettuce and sprouts giving body to a sandwich, you won't have to load up on the richer items. Here are some ideas to get started.

Hummus. The classic Middle Eastern spread (or dip) of pureed chick-peas and tahini (sesame butter). To keep fat content low, use more chick-peas and less tahini. If you use canned beans, drain off all the water—except what you'll need to get the blender to run—so your spread won't be too thin. Serve hummus or chick-pea puree in pita pockets with plenty of crisp, colorful vegetables.

Split-pea spread. Leftover split-pea soup or cooked split peas thicken in the refrigerator overnight for a fine sandwich spread. Add more seasonings if you like. This is especially good on hot toast; it almost melts.

Tofu spread. Tofu mayonnaise (see page 174) makes an excellent sandwich filler with lettuce or sprouts. Marinated tofu slices, heated or cold, work well in sandwiches, too. Marinate in two parts water to one part natural tamari soy sauce, then season with onions, garlic, or even hot-pepper sauce.

Vegetables. Thinly sliced cucumbers, grated carrots, alfalfa and radish sprouts, lettuce, and sliced tomato are great as stand-alone sandwiches. Try a mix of vegetables on a roll with a thin layer of tofu mayonnaise or Dijon-style mustard, or roll in a tortilla or chapati (you can use some steamed vegetables, too).

Tempeh. Tempeh makes a meaty sandwich, something like a pork tender-loin but lower in fat. Ready-made tempeh burgers and cutlets (some only need to be heated for one minute in a toaster oven) are in the freezer section at health food stores. Tempeh generously doused with barbecue sauce at the end of cooking and rolled in a tortilla burrito-style got rave reviews when a firefighter friend of mine fixed it at the firehouse—hardly a bastion of vegetarianism.

Fruit spreads. Remember jelly sandwiches from childhood? You can make them again using the fruit-only jams and preserves available at both grocery and health food stores. Or you can mix a dried fruit spread by gently simmering for one hour: Mix 4 cups of chopped dried fruit (prunes, raisins, and dates), 1½ cups water, ⅓ cup grated carrots, ⅓ cup lemon juice, and ½ teaspoon salt. Puree in your food processor (with a metal blade), and simmer again until it thickens.

Avocado. Make into guacamole by mashing avocados with chopped tomatoes and onions, garlic, and chili powder; add a squeeze of lemon juice to keep the avocado from turning brown, and salt to taste. Or slice thinly and combine with hot mustard, tomatoes, and sprouts. Cut the fat content in your favorite guacamole recipe by substituting cold, steamed broccoli for half of the avocado.

Burgers. Frozen, meatless burgers are now available at supermarkets and health food stores. My favorite are Boca Burgers—fat-free and absolutely scrumptious—but there are lots of choices; try them all.

Leftovers. Use the vegetarian loaves and burgers you've made for dinner. Many cookbooks include recipes for loaves and burgers made from grains like rice or oats with beans or chopped nuts, vegetables, and seasonings. Some of these can be mashed as is for next-day sandwiches. Others mix well with tofu mayonnaise. (Ready-made eggless mayonnaise is also available at health food stores. Check the labels; some are as high in fat as conventional mayonnaise, while others are reduced-fat. If you like mustard, you can sometimes use that as a substitute, too.)

Nut butters. Almond is my favorite. You can cut the fat content of any nut butter by mixing 1 tablespoon of it with 2 tablespoons of water and beating with a fork to emulsify them. You end up with more butter for the same amount of fat. Use nut butter on one slice of bread and fruit spread on the other.

Lettuce and shredded carrots provide a welcome, moist contrast to the dryness of the nut butter and bread. Sliced bananas are really good, too. Serve sandwiches with a lot of raw vegetables, a bowl of soup if you like, and an apple later if you're not quite satisfied. This is an ample and easy lunch—and when you bring it to work, I guarantee no one will say, "You must be on another diet."

BEAN CUISINE

WHETHER WE DON'T KNOW BEANS about something or it doesn't amount to a hill of them, beans are disparaged in metaphor and fact. Actually, this staple food comes in more than 50 varieties and has a 9,000-year history of cultivation that has made it important in nourishing and sustaining the human race.

Legumes are also a top choice food for the twenty-first century because they're full of fiber and minerals, provide quality protein without the drawbacks of protein from animal sources, and are in most cases very low in fat. They also keep well and are inexpensive. (Beans are cheap enough when you buy them, but when you consider that they swell with water during soaking and cooking, you're getting more satiety for the money. That's the opposite of meat, which shrinks when it's cooked, leaving you with less to eat than what you paid for. "You soak beans," said the most frugal cook I know. "They don't soak you.")

To cook beans, presoak them—with the exception of the smaller legumes, lentils, and split peas, which needn't be soaked. Place them in a large pot with two to three times their volume of water and let them stand overnight, for at least 8 hours.

Or to use the quick-soak method, bring the water to a boil and cook for 1 minute; turn off the heat, cover the pot, and allow the beans to stand for 1 to 2 hours. (The second method is supposed to reduce the likelihood that the beans will cause flatulence. Either way, discard the soaking water and cook them in fresh water.)

When you're ready to cook, bring the beans to a boil, then reduce the heat so you can cover the pot and let the beans simmer gently for the indicated amount of time.

If beans will be pressure-cooked, they do not require presoaking. Simply place them in the pressure cooker (three parts water to one part beans). Fill the cooker two-thirds full or less. Add 1 tablespoon oil to prevent foaming. Cover and bring to pressure. Begin timing when the gauge rocks. After the time is up, cool the cooker until pressure is down before removing the lid.

Cooking Times for Beans

Type of Beans	Stove Top (hr.)	Pressure Cooker (min.)
Black beans	1½–2	22–25
Black-eyed peas	1–1½	20
Chick-peas	2–3	40
Fava beans	2–3	40
Great Northern beans	1½–2	25
Kidney beans	1½–2	30
Lentils	½	N/A
Lima beans, small	1–1½	20
Lima beans, large	2	30
Navy beans	2	30
Pinto beans	1½–2	25
Soybeans	2½–3	30–35
Split peas	½	N/A

TOFU 101

Do you have some friends that you really had to get to know before you liked them? Tofu is like that. Once you get friendly with it, the odds are good that you'll be glad you did.

Tasteless on its own, tofu can take on the flavorings used with it to become a worthy pinch-hitter for such diverse and cholesterol-laden foods as ground beef, chicken, mayonnaise, cream cheese, sour cream, and eggs.

Made from soybeans, the richest in oil of all legumes, regular tofu weighs in at 53 percent fat per calorie. That's not low-fat when compared with other

Love-powered choices like bananas (3 percent), cabbage (7 percent), and kidney beans (4 percent). But when filling in for cream cheese (91 percent fat), hamburger (65 percent), or eggs (65 percent), there is a savings—not to mention that switching to tofu eliminates the other problems that come with using animal foods. And reduced-fat tofu is now available: White Wave makes tofu with a third less fat, and Mori-Nu makes 1% low-fat silken tofu.

Tofu is economical, easy to digest, and if precipitated with calcium sulfate, a good source of calcium. If you entertain guests a lot or if you miss animal foods or have a family to cook for that's resistant to change, tofu can make things easier.

By itself, tofu is like wet foam rubber, but you would no more eat it by itself and expect fine dining than you would stare at a blank canvas and expect to see fine art.

To become a Rembrandt with tofu, you first need to find it. Tofu is often in the produce department with the Asian vegetables. If you don't find it there, look in the dairy case where it's sometimes kept since it is so easily interchangeable with cottage, pot, farmer, feta, and ricotta cheeses. You can also locate tofu in aseptic packages so it needs no refrigeration or environmentally unpackaged for bulk sale at health food stores and Asian markets.

Tofu is often labeled according to its consistency: "extra-firm," "firm," "soft," and "silken" (very soft). Firm can be used for everything; soft is used for dips, sauces, and spreads. It gets confusing because silken tofu (the softest) can be labeled "firm" and "extra-firm." Don't worry about it. Think of silken as soft, whatever the label says.

Tofu must be kept in water. If you get it in bulk, store it in bowls of water in your refrigerator. If it comes in an unsealed carton (like cottage cheese), put it in fresh water when you get it home and refrigerate it that way. If your tofu is vacuum-packed, put fresh water on any leftovers after it has been opened. Change the water every two to three days.

Fresh tofu, when so cared for, will last 7 to 10 days in the refrigerator. (Vacuum-packed tofu lasts quite a while when refrigerated; check the date on the container.) In aseptic cartons, silken tofu lasts indefinitely. These containers generally only contain 10 ounces of tofu, so you don't need to worry about storing leftovers.

Try out these tasty, easy-to-make tofu fixings.

Salad dressing. Add to tofu in a blender a bit of lemon juice or cider vinegar, tamari (natural soy sauce), water as needed for the consistency you want, and whatever seasonings you fancy. My favorite is dried dillweed, but garlic and onion powder are always good, as is the spicy combo of curry and cumin.

Tofu mayonnaise. Drain tofu. Place in a blender or food processor 6 ounces tofu with 2 tablespoons lemon juice, 1 tablespoon oil, ½ teaspoon salt, ¼ teaspoon white pepper, and puree. If desired, add seasonings like onions and garlic—and pickles. (To lower fat content, omit the oil.)

Sandwich spreads. Mix mashed tofu with chopped vegetables like carrots and celery. Thin with tofu mayonnaise for spreading consistency.

Burgers. Mix mashed tofu with chopped or grated vegetables (onions, peppers, mushrooms) and some sesame or ground sunflower seeds. Use flour to make the mixture stiff enough to form burgers. Season with salt, tamari, basil, cumin, garlic, onions, or whatever. Bake or broil.

Tofu loaf. Use mashed tofu instead of ground beef in meat loaf.

Tofu steaks. Drain firm tofu. Slice in ½" thicknesses. Coat with flour and spices. Bake until crisp. (This is especially good if you marinate the tofu first with a mixture of half water and half tamari.)

Soup. Cut drained tofu into little squares and use to replace chicken in chicken soup. Use a chicken-flavored vegetarian broth mix from a health food store for the base. Simmer long enough for tofu to pick up the flavor.

Pudding or "yogurt." In a food processor, puree a block of tofu, about a tablespoon of honey or maple syrup, a teaspoon of vanilla, and a dash of salt. Adding carob powder makes a "chocolate" pudding. (If you're a real yogurt fan, cultured soy yogurt is sold ready-made at many health food stores. If you make yogurt yourself, that can be done with soy milk, too.)

THE GRANARY

Solid, centering whole grains are the staples of any healthful diet. Although they're filling and filled with a wide range of minerals and B vitamins, a full cup averages less than 2 grams of fat. Most grains can be cooked, sprouted (wheat and rye sprout particularly well), ground into flour, or made into pasta.

For hot breakfast cereals, add extra water if not topping with milk or soy milk. Cook with dried fruit for a sweetener, perhaps overnight in a slow cooker, or sweeten with a little maple syrup or date sugar. For side dishes, use like rice to make a bed for black beans or stir-fried vegetables. Use grains as an entrée, such as rice pilaf, millet stuffing for squash or peppers, or couscous served with steamed vegetables.

For grains ground into flour, use whole-wheat flour for yeast breads, and whole-wheat pastry flour for quick breads, cookies, and pie crusts. Use corn-meal for corn bread, muffins, and Johnny cakes and buckwheat for pancakes. Try rye flours for specialty baking or as an alternative to wheat for people with allergies.

Whole-wheat spaghetti and lasagna noodles can be found in supermarkets. Health food stores not only stock these but also pastas made from corn, rice, and buckwheat.

Whole grains can also be used in soups (barley is a natural here), in salads, like rice or pasta, or in desserts like rice or bread pudding. Your supermarket can provide you with whole-wheat bread (be sure the wrapper says 100 percent whole-wheat), whole-wheat pasta, brown rice, brown rice pilaf, wild rice, oatmeal, and whole-grain cold cereals like NutriGrain and shredded wheat. Health food stores have a vast array of whole grains as well as flours, pastas, and cereals made from them.

There are exotic grains to try like sticky-sweet amaranth and light, fluffy quinoa. And then there are the basics.

Brown rice. Long-grain brown rice cooks up in separate kernels to eat as is or use in pilafs; short-grain rice turns out sticky, good for croquettes and burgers or even pressed onto a pie plate as a fat-free crust for a tofu quiche or vegetable pie. Basmati is a gourmet rice from India with a nutty flavor and wonderful aroma. You can buy both brown and white basmati rice.

Buckwheat. Cook this like rice or as a hot breakfast cereal. Buckwheat (also called kasha) flour is fabulous for hotcakes.

Bulgur. Bulgur is cracked wheat, popular in Middle Eastern cooking, and the primary ingredient for tabbouleh, a wheat salad.

Corn. Although we don't tend to think of corn as a grain, we use cornmeal as such. Whole cornmeal—germ and bran included—is available at health food stores for use in hot cereal, bread, or polenta.

Millet. Tiny round grains that become puffy and delicate when cooked, millet can be used as a cooked cereal, stuffing, the base for burgers, or a side dish.

Oats. You can cook whole oats (called groats), but oatmeal—even the quick-cooking kind—is a whole grain, too. Use for breakfast, in baking, or as the base for veggie burgers. (You can eat extracted oat bran if you want, but you may as well get the bran with the rest of the oat as a whole food.)

Scotch barley. This is whole-grain barley; the refined kind is called pearl barley. Use in soups or as an alternative to rice.

Wheat germ. This is the nutritious heart of the wheat kernel. It's therefore not a whole (intact) food, and it's rich enough in oil to qualify as a rich relative. It is, however, a concentrated source of vegetable protein and vitamin E. When you are not using it, keep wheat germ stored in the refrigerator. And buy it toasted since raw wheat germ can go rancid very quickly. Wheat bran is sold separately, too, for dietary fiber, but the whole grain provides both the bran and the germ.

Whole wheat. Whole wheat berries may be cooked or sprouted as well as ground into flour for bread or pasta. Couscous is a quick-cooking wheat product that has been presteamed. Most of the couscous available is refined, but even if you can't find the whole-grain variety, this quick-cooking, company-pleasing grain deserves a place in your pantry.

Wild rice. An elegant addition to a special meal, this North American native can dress up an ordinary rice dish or make an exquisite stuffing for winter squash.

All these whole grains keep well. Store them in jars with tight-fitting lids; keep the jars in a cool, dry place. Refrigerate whole-grain flours and cornmeal.

When it comes to cooking grains, Nava Atlas, author of *Vegetarian Celebrations*, offers these simple suggestions: First, rinse the grains in a fine sieve (presteamed, rolled grains such as rolled oats don't require this). Toast them in a dry or lightly oiled skillet until the grains turn a shade darker and release a nutty aroma, then stir the grain into boiling water. Let it return to a boil and lower the heat, letting simmer, covered, until the water is absorbed.

Do not stir while the grain is cooking. (Note: Rolled oats, bulgur, and couscous do not require simmering; just turn off the heat and allow the grain to sit for the specified time.) If grains are too chewy at the end of cooking time, add another ½ cup of water for every cup of raw grain used; cover and simmer until water is absorbed.

Here are the cooking times for a few grains. They assume you're using two parts water to one part grain. Until you're used to whole grains, listen ahead of time to see if the simmering sound has stopped so you don't scorch a pot.

Grain Cooking Times

GRAIN	COOKING TIME (MIN.)
Brown rice	45
Buckwheat (kasha)	20
Bulgur, cracked wheat	15
Millet	40
Quinoa	15
Rolled oats	10
Wheat berries	60–90

FAT ZAPPERS

OUR BODIES DON'T REQUIRE EGGS or dairy foods or extracted oils, but for the kind of cooking we're used to, these foods seem essential. Vegetarian cookbooks can make you a masterful chef—or as close to that as you care to be—using no animal products and little oil. In my book *Get the Fat Out*, there are 500 such suggestions. For now, the following suggested substitutions should suffice. Most of these really zap the fat.

Eggs. For scrambled eggs, try some recipes for scrambled tofu or try the commercial product, Tofu Scrambler, found at health food stores.

In baking, substitute each egg with 1 teaspoon commercial egg substitute and 2 tablespoons water or use 1 tablespoon arrowroot powder, 1 tablespoon soy flour, and 2 tablespoons water. You can try this with 2 tablespoons flour, ½ tablespoon vegetable shortening, ½ teaspoon baking powder, and 2 tablespoons water; or blend 2 ounces tofu with the liquid called for in the recipe. Half a large mashed banana works, too.

In casseroles, burgers, and loaves, replace one egg with mashed potatoes or mashed avocados; or use moistened bread crumbs or rolled oats.

Milk. Try commercial soy milk (a low-fat variety), powdered soy milk (get soy milk powder, not soy flour), rice milk, or nut milk, like almond or cashew. (If you wish to continue using dairy milk, be sure it's free from additives.)

Cheese. Use mashed soft tofu (for ricotta), soy cheese (found at health food stores; fat content is comparable to dairy cheese without the cholesterol), or small amounts of miso or tamari (for salty flavor). Nutritional yeast or the rich relative tahini can substitute for Parmesan on pasta, or get soy Parmesan at health food stores. For cream cheese, use firm tofu blended with salt, dill, and lime juice to taste.

Shortening. In baking, substitute natural applesauce or prune puree (prune baby food works great) for the oil or butter you would otherwise use. You can also leave out up to one-third of the fat called for in the recipe without affecting the flavor, and pureed tofu can fill in for two-thirds of the remaining butter or oil.

Salad dressings. Blend vegetables and herbs with tomato and lemon juice, or cut oil in conventional recipes by half and substitute tomato juice or blended tofu. Also, try blending a small amount of nuts, seeds, or avocados with carrot, celery, or tomato juice—or with water, lemon, and savory seasonings to taste. Another option is to squeeze fresh lime juice on a salad to allow the taste of the vegetables to come through. Fresh lime or lemon juice and seasoned salt or herbal blend make for a sophisticated salad.

Oil. Use no-stick cookware to eliminate or cut down on oil (high-quality cookware with tight-fitting lids retains steam from vegetables, minimizing the amount of oil and other liquids required). Also spray-coat pans instead of using oil, or use other liquids like water, tomato juice, cooking sherry, apple juice, tamari (the reduced-fat kind works best for cooking), vegetable broth, or an oil/water combination (1 tablespoon oil to ⅓ cup water).

GOOD FOOD GADGETS

You don't need a kitchen filled with paraphernalia to create meals your body will truly appreciate. The important utensils will be some nice wooden spoons for stirring; a big bowl or two for mixing and for salads; some sharp paring knives; a couple of pieces of good, nonaluminum cookware with lids; a vegetable steamer; and either a blender or a food processor for making spreads, sauces, smoothies, cream soups, and the like.

Among the following good food gadgets, you'll find some you already own and some you may want to invest in. None is indispensable.

Blender. Ideal for shakes, smoothies, salad dressings, and sauces.

Citrus juicer. Inexpensive models, either manual or electric, are found in discount, department, and cookware stores. Fresh grapefruit, orange, and tangerine juices are exquisite.

Double boiler. Has two pots; one holds boiling water. Cooks gently—excellent for preparing grains such as millet or for reheating leftovers.

Food processor. Shreds, chops, mixes, and kneads. Helpful for making salads, dips, and purees.

Hot-air popcorn popper. For fat-free popcorn that you can season yourself with tamari, nutritional yeast (for a cheesy taste), or a dash of ground red pepper.

Mortar and pestle. Spices are best when freshly ground and this is the time-honored way to do it. (An electric coffee and spice mill is another option.)

No-stick cookware. Cut down on oil use by buying at least one high-quality, no-stick pan. Get one with a lengthy guarantee against chipping of the coating. It's also good to look for no-stick cookware that doesn't require the use of special utensils: Unless you live alone, someone is bound to use the wrong spatula. I like Millennium from Farberware. (Not all your cookware has to be no-stick. Have at least one piece—a Dutch oven or soup pot perhaps—in cast iron to maximize the iron in your diet.)

Rice cooker. This is a great boon for cooking perfect rice and for steaming vegetables. Plug it in and go away.

Pressure cooker. Popular in the 1950s, pressure cookers are back in more sophisticated models. Pressure-cooking is a real time-saver when beans are on the menu.

Salad spinner. This nifty contraption in cookware departments and gourmet shops will spin-dry salad greens in a jiffy.

Slow cooker. Let a slow cooker simmer up a one-pot dinner (soup, stew, chili, or homemade grain pilaf) while you're gone all day.

Sprouter. If you'd like to grow sprouts in a more sophisticated manner than the cheesecloth and jar technique (see page 164), there are perforated plastic trays, special bamboo bags, and a variety of other inventions for growing your sprout garden. Look for these at health food stores.

Vegetable juicer. Try a juicer with centrifugal force—it works great for extracting juices from carrots, greens, and all kinds of fruit. If you invest in a really good juicer (Champion is a good brand), you'll also be able to make soft-serve, fruit-based frozen desserts and fresh nut butters. Look for these in health food stores.

Vegetable steamer. You can get the vitamins and great taste that you would otherwise miss in cooked vegetables by buying a stainless-steel vegetable steaming rack for just a few dollars. Place it over boiling water in a pot with a tight-fitting lid. Put the vegetables on top and enjoy them a few minutes later. (An electric rice cooker works as a steamer, too.)

Wok. You can stir-fry in a large skillet, but a wok—an electric wok or one that you put on the stove—invites the frequent use of this healthful style of cooking. Look into a no-stick wok to keep oil use to a minimum.

You'll notice that I didn't mention microwaves. It's true that they save time and energy, and they can be a real help in cooking without added fats. If you already have one, you probably love it, so use it in good health. I don't recommend microwaves, however, because I don't think that microwaved food tastes as good as food cooked conventionally. As a practicing binge eater, I ate food no matter how it tasted. I don't have to do that today. Today I can have the best, even if it means waiting for it.

Also, I think that too much dependence upon microwaving—as well as on fast-food restaurants—can impede a food addict's recovery. Both quickly provide food—the ideal setup for a binge. When you cook beans and grains the old-fashioned way, taking your time is a given. When you're eating raw fruits and vegetables, there's no time spent fixing them, but plenty goes into chewing. Either way, a slow-down factor is built in. I have found through my own experience a good deal of value in this.

Also of value is seeing that your kitchen is a place that makes you smile. If yours is filled with unhappy memories of sneaking leftovers and midnight refrigerator raids, christen it as a new place, a friendly place supportive of your true needs and of loving yourself thin instead of coercing yourself that way. Hang up a picture that you treasure or quotations that mean something to you. You may want to treat yourself to new tableware. When I had a set of pottery dishes made that I had designed myself, I felt special. A bit of that feeling has stayed with each plate and bowl and mug. Every meal with these dishes feels like a special occasion, even though the set cost no more than ordinary stoneware.

Start with small things: Delight in your dishes or your herb plants or the inspirational needlework saying on the wall. You'll soon delight as well in how your eating has changed. It's all connected.

KITCHEN ECOLOGY

SIMPLY EATING NATURAL FOODS and leaving others behind takes some pressure off the Earth, but there are some other simple practices that you can undertake to lighten the planet's burden even more.

Try incorporating some of the following into your grocery shopping and food preparation routine.

Use cloth or string bags when you shop. If you have ever lived outside of the United States, you already know that this is a natural and pleasant way to shop. If you're without your cloth bags, paper is probably a better choice than plastic. Either way, reuse and then recycle them.

Buy in bulk when you can. Health food stores and co-ops often offer whole grains, flours, nuts, seeds, dried fruit, maple syrup, tofu, and other foods in bulk, allowing you to use your own refillable containers. When you have a choice, choose the product with the least packaging.

Store foods in jars you've saved or in other reusable containers. This will cut down on your use of plastic wrap and foil. You can also try cellulose storage bags made from plant fiber.

Save energy. You can do this by including lots of raw foods in your diet and by not cooking at the highest heat setting.

Compost your food scraps. This actually turns your garbage into rich soil that can be used in a garden or simply donated back to the Earth. It's easier than you think.

Forgo the disposable chopsticks at Chinese restaurants (or bring your own reusable pair). Disposable chopsticks are taking their toll on bamboo forests. In addition, keep a mug at the office instead of using Styrofoam, and suggest a switch to washable cups to your church or club groups.

Use cloth napkins. To make this practical, you won't want all your napkins lace-edged or made of heavy linen that needs to be ironed. Buy cotton or cotton/polyester bandannas, reasonably priced at camping equipment stores. One napkin a week per family member may be enough, but keep plenty on hand for guests, spills, and messy meals.

Allow clean dishes to air-dry. By doing so, you'll avoid the energy drain of your dishwasher's drying cycle. And whether you do your dishes by machine or with a pair of rubber gloves, use a detergent that's environmentally sound and tested without the use of animals.

Every concerned and loving action you take shows the Love-empowerment working in your life. Using a cloth bag instead of plastic is like making yourself a couple of baked potatoes instead of tearing into a bag of chips. Both show you care, and it's pretty difficult to practice genuine caring and to practice addiction at the same time.

RECIPES
• • • • • • •

The following recipes were created by my friend Sonnet Pierce, a young chef. She tested them and brought samples to my house for my approval. I can honestly tell you that every one of them is delicious, easy, and full of Love power.

Breakfast or Brunch

Fruit Juice Smoothies and Shakes

By using different fruit juices and fresh or frozen fruit, you can make endless varieties of delicious fruit shakes. Using frozen fruit makes shakes extra-thick and rich-tasting. Fruit is naturally sweet so no added sweetener is needed. Use whatever juice you like. Good choices are orange juice, pineapple juice, cranberry juice cocktail, and grape juice.

Basic Banana Smoothie

1   ripe banana
1   cup fruit juice

Combine the banana and juice in a blender. Blend on high speed until smooth.

VARIATIONS

Banana-Berry Smoothie: Add ¼ cup fresh berries, such as strawberries, blueberries, or blackberries.

Strawberry-Banana Fruit Smoothie: Use a frozen banana and add orange juice. Blend with 6 to 8 frozen strawberries. (To freeze bananas, peel and break the banana into pieces. Store in an airtight container.)

Makes 1 serving

Berry Shake

1   cup apple juice
6   large frozen strawberries
¼   cup frozen blueberries

Combine the juice, strawberries, and blueberries in a blender. Blend on high until smooth.

VARIATION

Try adding fresh or frozen peaches, mangoes, pears, and pineapple.

Makes 1 serving

Eggless French Toast

Some nice fat-free toppings for this French toast (and also the Banana French Toast) are maple syrup, honey, cinnamon, fruit jam, and applesauce.

⅓ cup soy milk, rice milk, or nonfat milk
2   teaspoons whole-wheat flour
¼   teaspoon vanilla
2   slices whole-grain bread

In a large shallow bowl, whisk together the milk, flour, and vanilla. Add the bread and allow to soak on both sides to absorb the batter.

Coat a large no-stick skillet with no-stick spray. Warm over medium-high heat. Add the bread in a single layer and cook until browned on both sides.

Makes 1 serving

Gingerbread with Honey–Glazed Pears

2   tablespoons honey
2   tablespoons orange juice
1   teaspoon vanilla
2   pears, peeled and thinly sliced
⅓ cup soy milk
1   teaspoon vinegar
½   cup molasses
2   tablespoons oil
1   tablespoon water
1   tablespoon applesauce
2   teaspoons egg substitute
1¼ cups whole-wheat flour
¼   cup unbleached white flour
1½ teaspoons powdered ginger
½   teaspoon ground cinnamon
½   teaspoon baking soda
½   teaspoon baking powder
⅛   teaspoon salt

Preheat the oven to 375°F. Lightly coat a 9" pie plate with no-stick spray.

In a small bowl, whisk together the honey, orange juice, and vanilla. Pour into the pie plate. Arrange the pear slices in the pie plate.

Place the milk in a medium bowl and stir in the vinegar. Allow to stand for 10 minutes to sour the milk. Whisk in the molasses, oil, water, applesauce, and egg substitute.

In a large bowl, stir together the whole-wheat flour, unbleached flour, ginger, cinnamon, baking soda, baking powder, and salt. Add the milk mixture and stir to moisten the dry ingredients; do not overmix. Pour into the pie plate.

Bake for 25 to 30 minutes, or until a wooden toothpick inserted in the middle comes out clean.

Let cool on a wire rack for 10 minutes. Run a knife around the edge of the cake and invert it onto a serving dish.

Makes 6 servings

Cranberry–Banana Muffins

¾ cup whole-wheat flour
½ cup unbleached white flour
2 tablespoons chopped pecans
2 tablespoons chocolate chips
1 teaspoon baking soda
½ teaspoon cinnamon
½ cup fresh or frozen cranberries
½ cup mashed banana
¼ cup honey
¼ cup water
1 teaspoon vanilla

Preheat the oven to 375°F. Lightly coat a 6-cup muffin pan with no-stick spray.

In a large bowl, whisk together the flours, pecans, chocolate chips, baking soda, and cinnamon. Stir in the cranberries.

In a medium bowl, whisk together the banana, honey, water, and vanilla.

Fold together the flour and banana mixtures until the dry ingredients are moistened. Do not overmix. Spoon into the muffin pan.

Bake for about 25 minutes, or until tops spring back when lightly touched.

VARIATION
Omit the chocolate chips and use blueberries in place of the cranberries.

Makes 6 muffins

Banana French Toast

⅓ cup soy milk, rice milk, or nonfat milk
⅓ cup mashed bananas
4 teaspoons whole-wheat flour
¼ teaspoon ground cinnamon
2 slices whole-grain bread

In a blender, blend together the milk, bananas, flour, and cinnamon until smooth. Pour into a large shallow bowl. Add the bread and allow to soak on both sides to absorb the batter.

Coat a large no-stick skillet with no-stick spray. Warm over medium-high heat. Add the bread in a single layer and cook until browned on both sides.

Makes 1 serving

Entrées

Spicy Oriental Soup

1   cup boiling water
6   dried shiitake mushrooms
½   cup thinly sliced onions
1   tablespoon grated fresh
    ginger
1   tablespoon minced garlic
1   teaspoon toasted sesame
    oil
1   cup julienned carrots
½   cup sliced button mush-
    rooms
2   cups vegetable broth
½   cup frozen or fresh peas
1   tablespoon reduced-
    sodium soy sauce
½   teaspoon chili paste
4   ounces angel hair pasta
2   tablespoons chopped fresh
    cilantro (optional)

Place the boiling water in a small bowl. Add the dried mushrooms. Let stand for 10 minutes. Remove the mushrooms from the water; reserve the water. Remove and discard the mushroom stems. Slice the caps and set aside.

In a large no-stick pot, combine the onions, ginger, garlic, and oil. Sauté over medium-high heat for 1 minute. Add the carrots, button mushrooms, and 2 tablespoons of the soaking water. Cook for 1 minute.

Add the broth, peas, soy sauce, and chili paste. Stir in the reserved mushrooms and remaining mushroom water. Cover and bring to a boil.

Break the angel hair in half. Add to the pot. Stir in the cilantro (if using). Cover and simmer for 5 minutes, or until the angel hair is tender.

NOTE: Chili paste is a very spicy sauce made from chili flakes and garlic. Look for it in Asian markets. If you don't have homemade vegetable broth, use a 14-ounce can and add enough water to make 2 cups. Or prepare broth from vegetable broth powder according to package directions.
Makes 2 servings

Vegetable Chili

This chili is great served with cornbread.

2   teaspoons oil
1   cup coarsely chopped
    onions
1   tablespoon minced garlic
½   cup finely chopped carrots
1   cup chopped mushrooms
2   tablespoons chili powder
1   teaspoon ground cumin
1   can (15 ounces) pinto or
    red beans
1   can (15 ounces) black or
    kidney beans
1   can (15 ounces) chopped
    tomatoes, with juice
1   cup corn
¼   cup finely chopped fresh
    cilantro

Warm the oil in a large no-stick or heavy-bottomed pot over medium heat. Add the onions and garlic and sauté for 5 minutes. Add the carrots and cook for 1 minute, then add the mushrooms and cook for 2 minutes. Stir in the chili powder and cumin.

Add the pinto or red beans, black or kidney beans, tomatoes (with juice), corn, and cilantro. Bring to a boil over medium-high heat. Reduce the heat to medium and simmer for 10 minutes.

NOTE: You may replace the canned beans with a total of 3 cups of cooked beans. In that case, it may be necessary to add a little salt and perhaps some molasses to increase flavor.

Makes 4 servings

Southwestern Salad

This entrée for two is also good as a side dish for four. If desired, replace the canned beans with 1½ cups of cooked black beans.

1   can (15 ounces) black
    beans, rinsed and drained
1   cup cooked long-grain
    brown rice
1   cup corn
½   cup finely diced sweet red
    peppers
¼   cup chopped fresh cilantro
2   tablespoons finely diced
    red onions
1   jalapeño pepper, finely
    chopped (wear plastic
    gloves when handling)
2   tablespoons lime juice

2   teaspoons minced garlic
1   teaspoon ground cumin
½   teaspoon ground coriander
    Salt (optional)

In a large bowl, toss the beans, rice, corn, red peppers, cilantro, onions, jalapeño peppers, lime juice, garlic, cumin, and coriander. Toss well to combine. Season with the salt (if using).

Makes 2 servings

Vegetable Stir-Fry

Serve over hot rice with additional soy sauce if desired.

1   tablespoon olive or canola oil
1   cup thinly sliced onions
1   tablespoon minced garlic
1   tablespoon finely chopped ginger
2   cups thinly sliced carrots
2   cups sliced mushrooms
2   cups sliced zucchini
1   cup sliced yellow summer squash
1   cup julienned sweet red peppers
2   tablespoons mirin
1   tablespoon reduced-sodium soy sauce
1   teaspoon cornstarch
1   tablespoon water

Warm the oil in a wok or large no-stick skillet over high heat. Add the onions, garlic, and ginger; cook, stirring constantly, for 2 minutes. Add the carrots; stir for 1 minute. Add the mushrooms, zucchini, squash, and peppers; cook, stirring frequently, for 3 minutes. Add the mirin and soy sauce; cook for 2 minutes, or until the vegetables are tender.

In a cup, dissolve the cornstarch in the water. Remove the pan from the heat and stir in the cornstarch mixture. Return the pan to the heat and cook for 30 seconds, or until the vegetables become glossy.

NOTE: Mirin is a sweet rice wine that can be found in Asian grocery stores. Any white wine or grape juice may be substituted.

Makes 4 large servings

Tofu Reubens

This is a popular sandwich at the Bluebird Cafe, a vegetarian restaurant in my hometown of Kansas City.

⅔   cup red wine
½   cup water
⅓   cup reduced-sodium soy sauce
1   package (16 ounces) extra-firm low-fat tofu, frozen and thawed (see note)
⅓   cup tofu mayonnaise (see page 174)
3   tablespoons ketchup
3   tablespoons sweet pickle relish
½   teaspoon honey
8   slices rye bread, sourdough bread, or pumpernickel bread
    Finely sliced red onions
    Thinly sliced Swiss cheese (optional)
1   cup sauerkraut, drained

In a large baking dish, combine the wine, water, and soy sauce. Cut the tofu lengthwise into ¼"-thick slices and add to the baking dish. Let stand for 30 minutes. Drain; reserve the marinade for another use.

Preheat the oven to 450°F. Lightly coat a baking sheet with no-stick spray. Add the tofu in a single layer. Bake for 20 minutes. Turn the pieces and bake for 10 more minutes.

In a small bowl, mix the mayonnaise, ketchup, relish, and honey. Spread on one side of each bread slice.

Divide the tofu among 4 of the bread slices; top with the onions and Swiss cheese (if using). Divide the sauerkraut among the remaining 4 bread slices. Arrange the bread in a single layer on a clean baking sheet. Broil for about 5 minutes, or until the cheese is melted and the sauerkraut is heated through. Assemble the sandwiches.

NOTE: To freeze tofu, just put the unopened package in the freezer overnight. Let thaw in the refrigerator. Freezing changes the texture of tofu, giving it a chewy consistency that works well in many recipes. Tofu mayonnaise can be purchased at health food stores; one brand is Nasoya.

Makes 4 servings

French-Bread Pizzas

This is a fast and easy dinner. For variety, substitute focaccia, pita, or sourdough bread for the French bread. You may also replace the pizza sauce with the Fresh Tomato Sauce with Garlic and Basil on page 197 (add a little tomato paste to thicken it). If you are in a real hurry, you can put the pizzas under a broiler, but watch them closely since they cook very quickly and burn easily.

1   loaf (1 pound) French bread
    About 1 jar (8 ounces) fat-free pizza sauce
    Toppings (see note)

Preheat the oven to 450°F.

Slice the bread ½" to 1" thick. Place on a baking sheet and bake for 5 minutes, or until lightly toasted.

Spread the sauce on the toasted bread and sprinkle with your choice of toppings. Bake for 10 minutes, or until the vegetables are cooked or the cheese (if using) is melted.

NOTE: Good toppings for the pizzas include sliced mushrooms, chopped onions, minced garlic, chopped red or green bell peppers, corn, shredded or thinly sliced zucchini, coarsely chopped spinach or arugula, chopped pineapple, marinated artichoke hearts, sliced olives, shredded low-fat mozzarella or soy cheese, crumbled feta cheese, and chopped fresh herbs.

Makes 4 to 6 servings

Nori Vegetable Rolls with Ginger Dipping Sauce

These are a vegetarian version of Japanese sushi, which can contain seafood but often doesn't.

VEGETABLE ROLLS

1¼   cups + 2 tablespoons water
½   cup white basmati rice
¼   teaspoon salt
2   tablespoons mirin
1   teaspoon seasoned rice vinegar
2   sheets of nori (8" × 7")
½   medium carrot, julienned

GINGER DIPPING SAUCE

1   tablespoon reduced-sodium soy sauce
1   tablespoon water
1   tablespoon lime juice
2   teaspoons finely minced ginger
1   teaspoon honey
½   teaspoon roasted sesame oil

To cook the rice: Combine the water, rice, and salt in a medium saucepan. Bring to a boil over medium-high heat. Reduce the heat to medium-low, cover, and simmer for 15 minutes, or until the water has been absorbed and the rice is tender. Remove from the heat and stir in the mirin and vinegar. Transfer to a large bowl and chill completely.

To make the dipping sauce: In a small bowl, combine the soy sauce, water, lime juice, ginger, honey, and oil. Set aside.

To assemble the vegetable rolls: Spread half of the rice horizontally along the 8" edge of one of the nori sheets. Make an even layer over the bottom two-thirds of the nori. Using half of the carrots, make a row horizontally across the middle of the rice. Roll tightly, starting on the side with the rice. Moisten the far edge of the nori with a little water so the roll will seal. (The carrots should be in the middle surrounded by a layer of rice with the nori on the outside.) Repeat with the remaining nori, rice, and carrots.

Using a sharp knife, slice off the rough ends. Cut the remaining roll into 1" rounds. Arrange the rolls on a platter with the cut side up. Serve with the dipping sauce.

NOTE: Nori are paper-thin sheets of dried seaweed. They can be found in Asian markets and health food stores. Mirin is Japanese rice wine; you may substitute white wine or white grape juice.

Makes 2 servings

Sides

Cornbread with Onions and Chili Peppers

2   cups cornmeal
½   cup whole-wheat flour
1   teaspoon baking soda
1   teaspoon baking powder
½   teaspoon salt
⅓   cup water
¼   cup molasses
1   can (15 ounces) creamed
      corn
1   can (4.5 ounces) chopped
      green chili peppers
1   teaspoon oil
½   cup finely chopped onions
¼   cup finely chopped sweet
      red peppers

Preheat the oven to 400°F. Lightly coat a 9" × 9" baking dish with no-stick spray.

In a large bowl, whisk together the cornmeal, flour, baking soda, baking powder, and salt.

In a medium bowl, whisk together the water and molasses. Stir in the corn and chili peppers.

Warm the oil in a large no-stick skillet over medium heat. Add the onions and red peppers. Sauté for 5 minutes, or until the onions are translucent. Add to the molasses mixture.

Pour the molasses mixture over the dry ingredients. Stir until the dry ingredients are moistened; do not overmix. Pour into the baking dish.

Bake for 35 minutes, or until the top is lightly browned and a toothpick inserted in the center comes out clean.

Makes 9 squares

Curried Cauliflower

½   teaspoon oil
½   cup thinly sliced onions
½   teaspoon brown mustard
        seeds
2   cups cauliflower florets
½   cup water
1   tablespoon lime juice
1–1½   teaspoons curry powder
        Salt (optional)

Warm the oil in a large no-stick skillet over high heat. Add the onions and mustard seeds. Sauté for 1 minute.

Add the cauliflower, water, lime juice, and curry. Reduce the heat to medium-high. Cook, stirring frequently, for 5 to 10 minutes, or until the cauliflower is tender. Add salt (if using).

Makes 2 servings

Hummus

If desired, serve with a lemon wedge so that extra lemon juice can be added to taste.
Hummus is good served as an appetizer with wedges of pita bread or with vegetable sticks.
It also works well as a sandwich filling; use whole-grain bread or a pocket pita and add
shredded lettuce, sprouts, cucumbers, tomatoes, red bell peppers, onions, or grated carrots.

1   can (15 ounces) chick-
    peas, rinsed and drained
2   tablespoons lemon juice
1   tablespoon tahini
    (sesame-seed paste)
1   tablespoon water
½–1 teaspoon minced garlic
¼   teaspoon ground cumin
    Pinch of ground red
    pepper

In a blender or food processor, combine the chick-peas, lemon juice, tahini, water, garlic, cumin, and pepper. Process for 2 minutes, or until smooth.

NOTE: If you're preparing your chick-peas from scratch, use 1½ cups cooked.

Makes 2 cups

Mashed Potatoes with Garlic and Basil

4   cups chopped potatoes
    (with or without skins)
2   cups water
1   teaspoon olive oil
¼   cup finely chopped onions
1   tablespoon minced garlic
¼   cup julienned fresh basil
    Salt (optional)
    Ground black pepper, to
    taste

Combine the potatoes and water in a large saucepan. Bring to a boil over high heat. Reduce the heat to medium and cook for 15 minutes, or until the potatoes are soft. Transfer the potatoes and water to a large bowl. Mash.

Warm the oil in a medium skillet over medium-high heat. Add the onions and garlic. Sauté for 2 minutes. Add to the bowl with the potatoes. Add the basil, salt (if using), and pepper. Mix well.

Makes 4 servings

Roasted Vegetables

These are good as a side dish or can be served over rice as an entrée. Tailor this dish to your tastes by adding other vegetables, such as red and green bell peppers, yellow squash, parsnips, winter squash, or any complementary vegetables in season.

¼ cup reduced-sodium soy sauce

2 tablespoons balsamic vinegar

1 tablespoon olive oil

1 tablespoon minced garlic

1 teaspoon dried thyme

1 teaspoon dried basil

Pinch of red-pepper flakes

Pinch of ground black pepper

¾ cup water

1 cup zucchini cut into 2" cubes

1 cup coarsely chopped red onions

1 cup small cauliflower florets

1 cup small broccoli florets

1½ cups potatoes cut into 1" cubes

1 cup carrots cut into 1" slices

1 cup sweet potatoes cut into 1" cubes

Preheat the oven to 450°F.

In a large bowl, mix the soy sauce, vinegar, oil, garlic, thyme, basil, red-pepper flakes, black pepper, and ¼ cup of the water. Add the zucchini, onions, cauliflower, and broccoli. Mix well. Let stand for 30 minutes. Using a slotted spoon, transfer the vegetables to a large baking dish; reserve the marinade. Spread the vegetables in an even layer.

Meanwhile, add the potatoes, carrots, and sweet potatoes to the marinade in the bowl. Mix well and let stand for 10 minutes. Using a slotted spoon, transfer the vegetables to another large baking dish; reserve the marinade. Add the remaining ½ cup water to the vegetables to prevent them from sticking.

Place both pans in the oven and bake for 20 minutes. Remove the zucchini mixture from the oven and set aside. Bake the potatoes for another 20 minutes.

Turn on the broiler. Broil the potato mixture for 10 minutes, or until browned. Stir well. Add the zucchini mixture to the potato mixture. Drizzle with 2 tablespoons of the remaining marinade. Toss lightly to mix. If needed, return the pan to the oven for a few minutes to reheat the zucchini mixture.

Makes 4 servings

Thai Slaw

½   cup water
3   tablespoons distilled white vinegar
1   tablespoon reduced-sodium soy sauce
1   tablespoon peanut butter
1   teaspoon honey
1½ teaspoons cornstarch
1   clove garlic, minced
¼   teaspoon crushed red-pepper flakes
4   cups thinly sliced green cabbage
½   cup grated carrots
¼   cup sliced red onions
2   tablespoons chopped fresh cilantro

In a small saucepan, combine the water, vinegar, soy sauce, peanut butter, honey, cornstarch, garlic, and red-pepper flakes. Whisk to mix well. Bring to a boil over medium-high heat. Cook for 1 minute, whisking constantly. Remove from the heat and let cool.

In a large bowl, mix the cabbage, carrots, onions, and cilantro. Add the dressing and toss to combine.

Makes 4 servings

Dressings and Sauces

Balsamic Vinaigrette

2   tablespoons balsamic
    vinegar
2   tablespoons orange juice
1   tablespoon olive oil
1   tablespoon stone-ground
    mustard
1   tablespoon water
2   teaspoons honey
1   teaspoon finely minced
    garlic
1   teaspoon reduced-sodium
    soy sauce
    Ground black pepper,
    to taste

In a large bowl, whisk together the vinegar, orange juice, oil, mustard, water, honey, garlic, and soy sauce. Add pepper.

Makes ½ cup

Creamy Herb Dressing

½   package (10.5 ounces)
    firm low-fat silken tofu
¼   cup chopped fresh parsley
¼   cup water
2   tablespoons cider vinegar
1   tablespoon honey
1   teaspoon olive oil
1   teaspoon stone-ground
    mustard
1   teaspoon nutritional yeast
    flakes
    Salt (optional)
    Ground black pepper, to
    taste

In a blender or food processor, combine the tofu, parsley, water, vinegar, honey, oil, mustard, and yeast. Process until smooth. Add the salt (if using) and pepper.

NOTE: This is a thick dressing. For a thinner dressing, add additional water or vinegar. Try other fresh herbs in place of all or some of the parsley, such as a mixture of basil, thyme, and oregano.

Makes about 1 cup

Creamy Vegetable Sauce

Serve this sauce over pasta or as a topping on baked potatoes.

1½	cups light soy milk or nonfat milk
¼	cup pureed winter squash or pumpkin
2	tablespoons mirin
1	tablespoon cornstarch
1	teaspoon nutritional yeast flakes
½	teaspoon salt
½	teaspoon reduced-sodium soy sauce
1	teaspoon oil
½	cup thinly sliced onions
1	teaspoon minced garlic
1	cup sliced mushrooms
½	cup fresh or frozen peas
1	teaspoon lemon juice
	Ground black pepper, to taste

In a blender, combine the milk, squash or pumpkin, mirin, cornstarch, yeast, salt, and soy sauce. Blend on high speed until smooth.

Warm the oil in a large no-stick skillet over high heat. Add the onions and garlic. Sauté for 5 minutes. Add the mushrooms and peas. Cook for 2 more minutes. Remove from the heat and stir in the milk mixture.

Return to the heat and cook over medium heat, stirring frequently to avoid lumps, for 5 minutes, or until thickened. Remove from the heat and stir in the lemon juice. Add pepper.

NOTES: Mirin is a sweet rice wine that can be found in Asian grocery stores. Any white wine or even white grape juice may be substituted. Nutritional yeast flakes are sold in health food stores and are not the same as baker's yeast, which cannot be substituted.

Makes 3 servings

Fresh Tomato Sauce with Garlic and Basil

This sauce may be used cold or warm (heat gently over low heat). Mix with hot pasta and garnish with basil leaves for a fast summer dinner.

2	cups chunked tomatoes
¼	cup coarsely chopped fresh basil leaves
3	tablespoons tomato paste
2	teaspoons minced garlic
	Salt (optional)
	Ground black pepper, to taste

In a food processor, combine the tomatoes, basil, tomato paste, and garlic. Process until pureed. Season with the salt (if using) and pepper.

Makes 2 servings

NINE
Love-Yourself Living

LOVE-POWERED LIFE IS A LIFE OF LOVE AND POWER. THE POWER doesn't come from the personal ego—defined, someone told me, as "edging God out"—but from the unlimited power of Love. When we talk about the power that heats our houses and runs our cars, the synonym we use for it is energy.

Adopting Love-powered principles, spiritually and physically, brings abundant energy into our lives. For one thing, there's more energy available from eating this way: Unrefined carbohydrates are known for fueling endurance athletes. And we can better take advantage of this greater energy because of the changes that have taken place in our thoughts and attitudes.

There are no rules to follow in order to live a love-based instead of a fear-based life. You can establish your own unique connection with universal Love. In general, though, this kind of life is defined by its ABCs—addiction-free, balanced, and compassionate.

Addiction-free. Spiritual renewal makes freedom from addiction possible. Sensible choices on the physical level are supportive of this. With daily dedication to your new way of life, you can expect not only freedom from the food fix but freedom from other imbalances that have held you back.

Balance. True balance comes about when generous portions of love and power are expressed harmoniously in a person's life. I think of it as working like this.

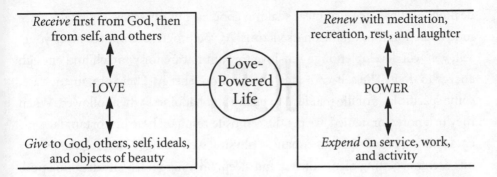

In practice, giving and receiving love become the same thing. Love can't be stored up like grain in a silo or coins in a jar, so the love you get must go out again. You become a conduit rather than a container. The more love you give, the more you're able to channel. It's the ultimate in recycling. Energy operates similarly. You renew your supply in quiet times with your Higher Power with rest, sleep, and having fun. Work that you love, exuberant activity, and doing some good in the world can also give energy back to you.

Compassion. Love and energy—giving and receiving, expending and renewing—enable lives to work. Lives that work best also reveal compassion. Compassion is the keynote of Love-powered eating and compassion, although interpreted in different ways, is central to any viable spirituality. Its literal meaning is "to feel with." You can "feel with" another because you've been hurt yourself and can empathize or because you've had compassion shown to you and you know how to pass it on. If you are a recovering food addict, you've experienced both the hurt of the addiction and then the compassion of your Higher Power and your supportive friends, even your own compassion for yourself as you became willing to live without the familiar crutch of excess food. Loving yourself thin expresses balance—a healthy, harmonious lifestyle—and compassion—empathy with others and having the love and energy to devote to them.

THE BALANCE OF HEALTHFUL LIVING

THERE ARE MANY WAYS IN WHICH BALANCE can be evident in a life, such as harmonious relationships, productive work, and responsible financial dealings. But balance also means taking good care of ourselves physically since food addiction robs that from its victims. As you progress in appreciating yourself, you will develop enough self-love to want to care for yourself and enough energy to do it. The self-care then creates more energy. There are, in any case, some specific laws of life that lead to health and happiness when followed. When they're ignored or denied, we get the opposite results. These important laws include: eating pure food that enhances physical well-being; doing regular, vigorous exercise; getting plenty of rest and sleep; breathing fresh air; drinking pure water; establishing a respectful relationship with the sun; and managing stress levels by developing peace of mind and emotional poise.

I used to think that if a person were spiritual enough, the physical self wouldn't matter. Now I see "spiritual" and "physical" as concentric circles, or colors in a rainbow, one fading into the next. The fact that there are natural laws to help us get more joy out of life is as close to a gift from God as anything I know.

When I was an active food addict, taking care of myself was near the bottom of my priority list. At times I slide back into some of my old ways, but the natural laws are always there for my benefit—and yours. Maybe I didn't get enough sleep last night or maybe I didn't exercise for five days straight. I can take a nap now. I can exercise today. So can you. And these healthy habits are self-propagating. Once you make room for them in your life, things don't seem right without them.

LOVE YOURSELF WITH ACTIVITY

EXERCISE IS GOOD FOR THE BODY, but it's even better for the spirit. Long before you observe that an increase in your activity level has blessed you with firmer muscles, greater stamina, and a more efficient metabolic rate, you will notice a heightened sense of well-being and self-worth. I know that this is true, even though I have a long history of detesting almost any endeavor capable of producing perspiration. I've come to appreciate how good moving my body can make me feel. Sometimes I love it. Sometimes I just go through the motions. When I start to truly dislike the exercise I'm doing, I know it's time to change it. That's because the body doesn't exercise alone; the mind comes along, too, and it also needs to enjoy itself.

It's not always easy because even the vocabulary that refers to physical activity makes it seem like chain-gang labor. *Exercise* sounds like *exertion.* People can be hospitalized for that. A *workout* doesn't sound like a great time either. My friend Dr. Douglas Graham, surely one of the fittest people I know, tells his patients, "I don't want you to work out. You work all day. In your free time I expect you to play."

Someone who is already fit like Dr. Graham might play as he does: trampolining in the backyard, hiking in the woods of Maine, skiing in Colorado, swimming in the Gulf of Mexico, taking 100-mile bike trips, or maneuvering through town on in-line skates with the agility of a carefree school kid on the first day of summer vacation. People who have been battling with their bodies for years, however, don't automatically equate exercise with play or pleasure. "Workout" seems like a most appropriate term, because hard exercise taken too soon can feel like work, drudgery even, and for someone with a very low level of fitness, demeaning drudgery.

Most of us who were overweight as children have horrible memories about sports and athletics. We were chosen last for teams—and grudgingly at that. We were called names by our classmates and chided by physical education teachers, and we experienced real suffering doing what everyone else apparently regarded as fun. We rubbed sores on our thighs when we tried to run. Our throats burned as we gasped for air, hoping to keep up in the sprint or make it to the bases. And the emotional pain of being seen in a swimsuit or showering after gym class was as acute as any physical discomfort.

Specific, conscious memories can fade, but those painful feelings attach themselves in our minds to the entire realm of exercise and participatory sports. It's no wonder that even after we're grown up, many of us regard exercise as a threat. People who were not heavy in childhood but gained extra weight later can have another problem. They remember how good it once felt to run and jump and dance. Thinking that they can't do these things now makes them feel sad and old when decades of promise still lie before them.

But you can move your body—and enjoy doing it. Whether you were heavy as a child or not, regardless of your current weight or age, you will be a happier as well as a fitter person when you start to use your muscles regularly and pleasurably. Remember that we're talking about a loving approach to diet and to life. A "no pain, no gain" philosophy does not fit here. Taking it slow is not only advisable, it is mandatory.

For exercise to do for you all that it can, it has to become an integral part of your life. It's not to be used like some willpower diet just until you get thin. And it's not to be put off until after you're thin, after you save the money to join a health club, or after you get around to putting air in your bicycle tires at some nebulous future point. You do it today because your body is a living organism that craves movement. Look at toddlers and puppies: The urge to be active is innate. If you think that urge in you is dead, it isn't. It's only sleeping. Don't try to jolt it awake with 50 pushups and a 5-mile run. Nudge it gently.

If you are over 40, are overweight, or have health problems requiring a special exercise regimen (diabetes, high blood pressure, heart disease, and arthritis are among these), by all means work out your fitness program with a knowledgeable physician. In any case, begin slowly. This is not just because it's easier on your heart and your joints to build up gradually but also because if you don't love what you're doing, you're likely to leave it. Sporadic exercise—a week here, a weekend there, a long layoff, then a ski trip—does almost nothing for a body and is an open invitation to injury.

Ideally, you exercise because you love yourself and the activity. It is not necessary that you be a distance runner, a belly dancer, or a power lifter. What is necessary for a fit and healthy life is that you be active enough for your body to function optimally. The general rule for accomplishing this is a minimum of 20 minutes of aerobic exercise three times a week. Aerobic (oxygen-utilizing) exercises are those that can be done for prolonged periods, like walking, running, swimming, skating, cycling, rowing, or dancing. This type of exercise is believed to be of particular benefit to the heart and circulatory system, to revive a sluggish metabolism, and to help normalize an unreasonable appetite.

Aerobic activity is not the only sort of useful motion that exists, however. The luxurious limbering and stretching of yoga and modern dance promote youthful flexibility, and strength-building exercises like weight training can sculpt a body to its best and provide it with more lean tissue. Lean tissue is a metabolism booster.

If you're approaching exercise as a beginner, choose something that you think you'll like. If you're a loner, you may want to invest in a stationary bike or a treadmill. If you love the outdoors, you'll probably prefer to jog or cycle whenever the weather permits and schedule some enjoyable backup activity when it doesn't. If you're gregarious, you'll like taking classes or belonging to a gym. Don't expect your basic personality to change to fit some arbitrary exercise plan: It won't.

I, for example, live with a state-of-the-art treadmill. Am I using it? Not on your life. I'm at my desk communicating with you. I'm a communicator, one of the gregarious types. When I'm at the health club, I exercise (and communicate) energetically; if I had to exercise at home by myself, I would probably be suffering from advanced muscle atrophy. But since exercise is now an integrated part of my lifestyle, one that I miss when deprived of it, I would find some sociable exercise even if I couldn't belong to a gym. Maybe I'd invite people over to work out to an aerobics video three mornings a week or join a group that walks at the mall. Whatever it took, I would get my needs met, both my personality's need for contact with others and my body's need for physical activity.

Some of the ways you may wish to meet your inborn need for activity are:

Walking. Where do you like to walk? Through the woods? Along country roads? I love to walk in cities. From my point of view, the best part of being in New York City or Chicago or San Francisco is walking all over, feeding pigeons, looking in shop windows, exploring parks and cathedrals, and taking in the sights and sounds and energy of the city. When walking is your activity of choice, you can do it anywhere, and the only equipment it takes is a pair of sturdy, well-fitting walking shoes. If you don't like the idea of exercise, see your walking as simply taking a walk. My friend Robin calls people she knows and asks if they would like to walk with her, the way we would more often ask someone out for a drink or a meal. It's a really charming invitation.

Or walk alone. Then you can vary your pace to suit yourself. Your walking may evolve into jogging or speed-walking. On alternating days when you aren't looking for a bona fide aerobic workout, you may forgo speeding things up in favor of slowing them down. Then you can treat yourself to the serenity of meditative walking.

Swimming. The problem with swimming is the bathing suit. The real difficulty there lies not so much in the suits or how we look in them but how we think that we ought to look in them. Self-acceptance may never have a tougher test than the swimsuit competition—the one in which the beautiful reality that you are today is challenged by advertising's persuasive image of how a body is supposed to look. Your growth in self-love will help you win in that internal swimsuit competition, and your new lifestyle will bring your body to its ideal state of health and fitness. Swimming—suit and all—can be part of that.

When you swim, you feel light. Movements that would be labored if not impossible on land can be almost effortless. Swimming is an aerobic activity, yet it's also relaxing and conducive to contemplation. One winter I belonged to a health club equipped with an indoor/outdoor pool. I went in the mornings before work and felt incredibly accomplished when I showed up at the office knowing that I had been swimming while snow fell all around me. If you plan to swim, be sure that the pool you choose has an atmosphere that's really pleasing to you. If the hours there aren't convenient, if the water is too cold, or for that matter, if the staff is too cold, look elsewhere.

Cycling. Bicycling appeals to my practical nature since it can be efficient transportation as well as aerobic exercise. If you can possibly use a bike for some of your commuting needs, I can almost guarantee that your life will change for the better in ways you might never have imagined. If you bike to work, your status in the company will improve even before your next promotion. That's because people are awed when someone actually demonstrates self-sufficiency, and getting to the job via person-power is self-sufficiency of the highest order. My fondest memory as a peddling commuter is whizzing past the bus I would otherwise have taken every morning. Of course, the same hill that enabled me to fly past a bus on my morning route had me huffing and puffing in the evening. It was worth it.

Biking is excellent for the not-yet-in-shape because you can pace it to your fitness level from short trips on flat land to touring the Rockies. It helps to have a comfortable bicycle. The balloon-tire single-speed bike in the garage can provide you with a workout, but a bike with gears lets you compensate for hills and feel less fatigued.

Some day you may want to race or enter a triathlon or get into mountain biking. Then again, you may prefer to pedal a stationary bike in your own family room while you watch a sit-com on the television. You get what you're after either way.

Aerobics classes. If you always wanted to be in the chorus line of a Busby Berkeley musical, you'll love aerobics classes. They provide the opportunity for anyone to dance, regardless of her number of left feet. (I say "her" because aerobics classes are overwhelmingly female, but men who summon the nerve to try it have a really good time. And, as you may imagine, the two or three men in a class of women are very popular.)

My preference is for low-impact aerobics, which minimizes stress on the joints. Just because it's called low-impact, however, does not mean that a class is low-intensity. It can be quite intense and call for a well-developed state of fitness to be fun or, for that matter, effective. If a session is too difficult, it won't even be aerobic for you: You'll overexert and your heart rate will go beyond the aerobic training range—the point at which you're breathing hard enough to know that you're exercising but not so hard that you can't comfortably carry on a conversation. Don't sign up for any classes you can't try out first. If a class is too tough and the instructor won't help you tone it down, find another.

Sometimes YMCA's and health clubs offer classes geared to beginners or senior citizens. I took a seniors' class when I was still in my thirties because it was the only one that fit my schedule. Along with weight training, that class put me at my highest level of fitness ever. It was easy enough to be fun. I enjoyed it, so I rarely missed a session. The teachers were friendly and down-to-earth. The participants encouraged each other. These are important qualities for you to look for in an aerobics program. Teachers should also be certified to teach aerobics and the facilities should accommodate this kind of class, with enough room for every student and a shock-absorbing floor to protect your knees and ankles as you exercise. Finally, music is an integral part of dance-aerobics. If you like the music, chances are you'll stick with the class—and you'll hum a lot the rest of the time.

Weight training. Working with weights can make profound changes in how your body looks in a short time. Even more meaningful is how differently people start to regard themselves when they've been involved with weight training for a while. Instead of feeling weak or routinely taking the victim's role, a person who trains with weights notices a feeling of competence and confidence after only a few weeks. Strong people tend to feel strong, inside and out. You can set up a home gym, but a well-equipped club can provide you with safety, instruction, and moral support. Working with a personal trainer who really cares about your progress can make up for all the unkind gym teachers you ever had. Verbal support like, "One more lift: I know you can do it!" can work wonders, not just for your deltoid or triceps muscles but for your sense of self.

Yoga. If you don't love your body yet, yoga can help you get to that point silently and surely. Hatha yoga—physical postures and breathing techniques—is thousands of years old. It comes from the Indian subcontinent, but its benefits are not confined to a single country or belief system. Its slow movements, coupled with controlled breathing, result in a calming of the body and mind. Yoga develops flexibility of the entire body, particularly the spine, and is believed to have various therapeutic applications.

Yoga was the first step I took in learning to love and care for myself. It put me in touch with my body. I had long tried to forget that I had a body since I always judged it as being fat or flabby or not measuring up in some other way. In yoga, I began to experience my body in a nonthreatening environment. The first thing I noticed was that I did have some natural flexibility. My self-image was then able to incorporate for the first time a positive trait that didn't have to do with being intelligent or having a good personality but one that belonged to my physical self. I also found my yoga teachers to be kind and patient. I remember one teacher saying, "Don't worry about changing your diet. Allow your spirituality to grow and that will change your diet."

If you're interested in yoga, visit a class and get a sense of it. Instructors of traditional hatha yoga are adept at the slow, calming style of this ancient discipline. There are other styles of yoga that are rougher, even harsh. Some people do well with these, but if you don't feel better when you leave a yoga class than when you came, find another. Just as you'll need a soft mat to protect your back when you do yoga, your class should have an atmosphere that's like a cushion. After all, you're loving yourself to thinness, so you may as well love yourself to fitness, too. When you approach your chosen physical activity or activities in this way, you guard against addictive exercise while incorporating healthy movement into your life.

LOVE YOURSELF WITH REST

O UR SOCIETY DOES NOT THINK TOO HIGHLY of rest and sleep. Resting is seen as laziness and sleep as a wasteful, albeit unavoidable, time expenditure. We fit these in because we would collapse if we didn't.

Pushing ourselves—even with stimulants like caffeine—is accepted. Whether the goal is the honor roll or the executive suite, we give our work all we've got. That's fine up to a point, until we realize that "all we've got" is, physically, all we have. What we're talking about, this intangible substance that propels us, is vital energy. In yoga this life force is called *prana*. In martial arts it's referred to as *chi*. Whatever we call it, it has to be regularly replenished. The natural way to do that is with adequate rest and sleep.

How much is adequate? Whatever is enough for you to feel good. Most adults require at least 7 hours of sleep per night. One way to find out what's right for you is to stop using an alarm clock. Try this on the weekends first so you won't be afraid of being late for work and wake up at 3:00 A.M. wondering if you've overslept. After you've done this for a while, you'll discover that you have an exceedingly efficient internal clock. When you awaken to it, you'll be refreshed. Even confirmed night people become much more tolerant of mornings when the clock radio is silenced and the internal clock takes over. (Don't worry about missing music in the morning: Do this and you'll sing.)

If you have had trouble sleeping, many of the lifestyle changes recommended here may be helpful in that regard. People who have considered themselves chronic insomniacs have found that simply cutting out caffeine, not just in the evening but all the time, solves the problem. Exercise is also valuable. The body strives for balance (the fancy word for that physiological balance is homeostasis), so exercise naturally invites rest and sleep as its balancers. Meditation, too, produces the deep relaxation that encourages peaceful sleep.

Sleep isn't the only kind of rest we need. We are supposed to rest whenever our bodies give us tired signals. We've misinterpreted these signals in all sorts of ways. For most food addicts, tired feels like hungry. The message can also reach our brain sounding like, "It's time for a cup of coffee," "Work harder, lazy!" or "Everything is irritating me and I'm about to explode." The next time you get any of those messages in the midst of a busy day, take a minute to examine them. Behind the hunger or the caffeine craving or the irritation might just be your body asking for a catnap, a walk outdoors, a brief conversation with another person, or just a switch from filing to typing or vice versa.

When you have sizable chunks of rest time, be sure that your rest is really restful. Watching the news or a murder mystery on television isn't an athletic event, but it's not resting either. You can rest with a book, but you can rest more fully while lying in a hammock watching the clouds. You can rest in a reclining chair listening to soothing music. You can rest by daydreaming, contemplating, or unwinding in a bath scented with lavender or juniper. Massage can also be sublimely restful. Honor your uniqueness by discovering those restful pursuits that make you say, "Ahh."

LOVE YOURSELF WITH FRESH AIR

T AKE A DEEP BREATH. IT FEELS GOOD, doesn't it? Do it again and really blow out on the exhalation. It's a great feeling, both relaxing and energizing at the same time. Our breath is our lifeline, although we seldom pay it any conscious attention. We don't have complete control over the quality of the air we breathe, but there are some actions we can take to breathe a little easier.

If you smoke, stop. Certainly this is a tall order because nicotine addiction is a powerful one. Whether you want to deal with your overeating or your smoking first or whether you want to make both of those changes simultaneously is up to you. Smoking is generally regarded as a more rapid form of suicide than binge eating, but to get all the life you're entitled to, get rid of both. Do not worry about eating more when you quit smoking. You are committed to loving and caring for yourself—your whole self. As long as you cling to any crutch to stay thin, especially a potentially fatal crutch like cigarettes, you won't know the freedom of total recovery.

Get the help you need to quit. The American Cancer Society and the American Lung Association both offer programs to help smokers become ex-smokers. Seventh Day Adventist churches and the hospitals affiliated with them offer smoking-cessation programs. (Their suggestions include cutting out red meat and caffeine to lessen the craving for nicotine, so you would be ahead of the game.) Smokers Anonymous, which uses the Twelve Steps, is growing. The most important thing is that you don't give up.

Even nonsmokers have to battle smoking. This means, don't breathe someone else's secondhand or sidestream smoke. It's hazardous to your health as well as uncomfortable. I've never been a smoker, but it used to be that when a hostess at a restaurant asked, "Smoking or nonsmoking?" I'd say, "It doesn't matter." That translates as "I don't matter." But I do, and you matter just as much. You have rights. Stand up for them. This is especially true in your own home. If no one in your family smokes, it's my opinion that you don't need an ashtray. Your home may not be a castle, but it doesn't have to smell like a pool hall either.

Open windows, especially at night. We go so nonchalantly from central heat to central air that we forget there's another kind of air—the fresh kind. Letting some in will revive your spirits and having fresh air circulating in your bedroom at night can become a positive habit you'll always keep. Expect your quality of sleep to improve once you try this. (If it's winter, just open a window a little and use an extra blanket.)

Give your household air a pollution check. Look in the Yellow Pages under "Environmental Services" or "Air Pollution Control" to find a company that can inform you about your indoor air quality. They'll check for pollutants such as radon (airborne particles of radium from decaying rock that are believed to cause lung cancer), formaldehyde (a suspected carcinogen that can come from carpets, paneling, and formaldehyde-foam insulation), and carbon monoxide as a combustion byproduct of fuels, as well as for dusts and molds that can aggravate allergies. If problems are found, there are ways (other than moving) to remedy them. Getting your air ducts cleaned every couple of years is a good idea, too.

Don't be a domestic polluter. Improve your home's air quality by using environmentally sound household cleaners, commercial or homemade, in place of harsh chemicals. Fumes from these (whether you can smell them much or not) end up in the air you breathe. (Just as using strong chemicals can decrease your air quality, having houseplants around can increase it by providing fresh oxygen.)

Do what you can to curb pollution in your community: Plant trees. Support clean air legislation. Become involved in local pollution-control campaigns or back the people who are involved.

Treat yourself to "gourmet air" when you can. Gourmet air is the best there is—the sort you'll find in the mountains, in the woods, and at the shore. Nature's most beautiful spots are also first-rate air purifiers.

LOVE YOURSELF WITH WATER
• •

You CAN LOVE YOURSELF WITH WATER externally and internally. We take baths and showers for granted, but have you noticed lately that it feels terrific to get clean? A shower is an invigorating experience; a bath is relaxing. Either one can be made special by using products that smell good and feel good. There's no reason why men as well as women can't treat themselves to scrumptious scents. The products that incorporate aromatherapy—oils that not only smell wonderful but are believed to have subtle, therapeutic effects on the mind and body—are not gender-exclusive.

Baths call for a lot more water than showers do. If you're going to take a bath, make it worth the water. Set aside enough time to really enjoy the process. Take the phone off the hook or, if your answering machine is playing receptionist, turn down the ringer so your thoughts won't turn from your relaxing bath to "Who could that be?" (I've left a hot, fragrant tub to take a phone call that turned out to be a talking computer that wanted me to buy aluminum siding. Today, I'd give the bath priority.)

Do a little more with your bath than you think you deserve. It's good practice in stretching your ability to love yourself. Does it seem outrageous to you to light incense in the bathroom or bathe by candlelight? Do it anyway. There's no better place to begin than in the privacy of the bath. (This is also a good place to start appreciating your body. Look at it kindly, touch it with care, and talk to your body. It will respond.)

To love yourself internally with water, you'll need to obtain the purest drinking water you can. As hard as it is to believe, our bodies are more than half water, and the water we drink, like the food we eat, really does become us. You have no doubt read that it's good to drink lots of water (six to eight 8-ounce glasses a day according to most health experts). We do need a great deal of water for our systems to function properly. If you're eating an abundance of fresh, raw fruits and vegetables, though, these are largely comprised of water, so you don't have to drink all the water you need. You'll be eating some of it. Generally, thirst is a fully efficient guide to when you should drink. The trick is answering that body signal with water instead of a soft drink or a beer.

Then there's the matter of what kind of water to drink. For most of us, tap water is not the best choice. Agricultural runoff and other pollutants enter the groundwater, which is then treated with chlorine in city water systems. Chlorine kills germs, but it does nothing to mitigate chemical pollutants. It is, in fact, a potent chemical itself.

Intelligent options include purchasing bottled water (in glass containers if possible; plastic can leach into the water) or a home distillation unit. Use pure water for preparing all your foods and beverages, for making ice cubes, and for drinking.

LOVE YOURSELF WITH SUNLIGHT
• •

UNLIGHT—ENOUGH BUT NOT TOO MUCH—is a necessity for plants to grow, for children to grow, and for life to exist on Earth. We've been well warned about the dangers of excessive sun exposure. Particularly at this time in history when the thinning of the ozone layer is causing more radiation from the sun to permeate the Earth's atmosphere, baking your body in the sun is not just a cosmetic indiscretion; it could lead to skin cancer. Nevertheless, you can also drown in water, exercise to the point of exhaustion, or rest so much that you never get anything done. This doesn't mean that you should never bathe, exercise, or rest. We need sunlight. We simply have to approach it with intelligence and respect.

A fascinating book on the subject is *Sunlight* by Zane R. Kime, M.D. In his book, Dr. Kime cites scientific studies demonstrating the beneficial effects of exposure to sunlight in a variety of medical conditions. Unlike many of his colleagues who tell their patients to avoid the sun as much as possible, Dr. Kime recommends modest but regular sun exposure geared to individual skin type and the climate in which a person lives.

One of his most fascinating contentions—one he documents from scientific literature—is the sunlight/nutrition connection. He writes: "Unless one has a proper diet, sunlight has an ill effect on the skin. This must be emphasized: Sunbathing is dangerous for those who are on the standard high-fat American diet or do not get an abundance of vegetables, whole grains, and fresh fruits.

Those on the standard high-fat diet should stay out of the sun and protect themselves from it, but at the same time they will suffer the consequences of both the high-fat diet and the deficiency of sunlight." Dr. Kime recommends a vegetarian diet of unrefined foods with ample representation from those foods rich in vitamins C and E and beta-carotene, abundant in yellow and leafy green vegetables.

When you and the sun get together, use your head to give the best to your body. Here are some suggestions: Appreciate what sunny weather does for your disposition. When a day is really glorious, don't shut yourself off from it. Have breakfast on the patio or take a walk during your coffee break. Take advantage of every beautiful day. For safety in the sun, remember Dr. Kime's dietary suggestions and stick with natural foods, avoiding animal fats and most extracted oils.

Remember, there's a difference between spending time outdoors on a bright morning or afternoon and lying on a beach at midday. One is safe and healthful, the other foolhardy. When you approach the sun, follow the "baby rule." You wouldn't put a baby out in the noonday sun, but you wouldn't keep a baby indoors all the time either. Baby yourself.

LOVE YOURSELF WITH PEACE OF MIND
•••••••••••••••••••••••••••••••••••

THE BODY AND THE EMOTIONS are intimately connected and interdependent. Many of the physical practices we've alluded to in this section—enjoying sunlight, getting enough rest, energizing with exercise—are natural antidepressants. Eating whole, natural foods also fosters emotional well-being because the brain is part of the body nourished by the foods we eat. Sharp highs and lows in blood sugar levels precipitated by eating refined sweets can cause mood swings.

Just as positive and negative physical actions can positively and negatively affect our emotions, emotions can in turn affect us physically. We've all experienced this mind/body interaction: feeling our faces flush when we're embarrassed, getting sweaty palms or butterflies in the stomach when we're nervous, or salivating at the very thought of sucking a lemon or biting into a sour pickle. Most overeaters have also seen that bouts of compulsive eating can be tied to anger, fear, or some unidentified emotional malaise.

The science of psychoneuroimmunology deals with how the mind affects the body. It presents convincing evidence that love, joy, laughter, gratitude, and hope can prevent and may even help cure disease. The implication is that happiness doesn't just feel good; it does good.

No one could be happy all the time if that meant being elated, giddy, and ecstatic nonstop. No rational person would expect to sustain such an emotional peak. Besides, we couldn't if we wanted to: Those extremes come in response to external events—events over which we have little (if any) control. The kind of happiness we can depend on is contentment. It's not exciting like elation, giddiness, and ecstasy, but it's only minimally dependent upon outside happenings. We learned earlier that the body seeks to maintain homeostasis (balance). The mind does, too. When your mind is in a state of balance, contentment is commonplace. You can call it serenity, equanimity, emotional poise, or peace of mind. By any name, it's great stuff.

Certainly things can happen in life that could shake the serenity of a saint, but balanced people have a high contentment quotient and they quickly regain a comfortable level of calmness. This occurs in spite of what is going on around them. Besides, it's not usually some major calamity that interferes with our happiness. "Nobody has ever tripped over Pikes Peak," my friend Mary Beth used to tell me. "It's the little stuff that will get you."

The starting place for dealing with this little stuff (and the more serious challenges) is the same place you started at in dealing with your food addiction: surrender. Leave the outcome up to God.

Surrendering the outcome doesn't mean that we do nothing to help ourselves. An image shared with me was that of seeing our Higher Power as an orchestra conductor and ourselves as musicians. Musicians certainly don't "do nothing." They make beautiful music. But they do it under the direction of a conductor. Like those musicians, we're at our best when we do what we can and refrain from doing what we can't.

Two things we cannot do are change other people and avert natural law. Who would try anything that ridiculous? We would. We have. We've tried to change people by getting thinner (so he or she would be attracted to us), by working harder (so our bosses would like us better), and by being more self-sacrificing (so our children would appreciate us). We've attempted to get around natural law, too—usually the laws of physiology: "This box of cookies doesn't

count because I'm starting a diet tomorrow" may sound familiar, as might praying to lose weight without giving up the food fix. When we stop trying to change
others and circumvent the laws of nature, we can get busy with those actions
that are ours to take on our own behalf. These actions bring us more peace of
mind. They include:

> Doing all we can to live in accordance with what we believe to be the will
> of our Higher Power. Peace Pilgrim, a remarkable woman who taught that
> inner peace was the prerequisite for world peace, was fond of saying, "Live
> up to the highest light you have, and more light will be given you."

> Allowing ourselves to be changed. Many of us have been self-help experts.
> We've done everything to change ourselves. Allowing ourselves to be
> changed is something else. The phrase that fits here is, "Let go and let
> God."

> Performing the next task that is ours to do. The Buddhists have a lovely
> concept called dharma. It translates roughly as duty. Every person has a
> dharma, a calling or purpose, distinctly his or her own. We can work our-
> selves into a frenzy trying to do someone else's dharma, but when we're
> committed to finding and doing ours, a peace comes with it.

> Treating ourselves with respect and expecting the same from others. We
> show self-respect with respectful thoughts about ourselves and respectful
> actions toward ourselves. Healthy self-respect does not allow us to play
> roles like victim and martyr. We learn to detach emotionally or separate
> physically from harmful relationships.

> Learning to accept or change negative circumstances. Sometimes we need
> to temporarily accept a not-so-perfect situation, like a job that doesn't use
> our skills or an apartment with noisy neighbors, and acknowledge that it
> can be changed later. We learn to do both these things by giving our high-
> est good a priority. In fact, changing and accepting are the only healthy
> options in any situation. We all know that deep down. That's why "The
> Serenity Prayer" has such universal appeal.

This last one especially is not easy because we've grown accustomed to trying to control things. Even the phrase, "trying to control things," makes my jaw tighten and my shoulder muscles tense. A change in vantage point is needed for peace of mind to become natural for us. Most people can't make the shift without some help. The Twelve Step programs are excellent resources for this help because the steps heal emotionally as well as physically and spiritually. Practicing them to recover from a food addiction (or from any addiction) brings about a noteworthy degree of emotional poise and inner peace.

In addition to a support group, professional counseling can be useful. If you had counseling when you were involved in food addiction (whether you were practicing compulsive eating or compulsive dieting), it may have seemed like a waste of money and time. Do consider it again if you feel the need. You're bound to find the experience far more meaningful when you enter it without the impermeable barrier of active addiction between you and the help being offered. Remember that the therapist works for you. You have to like this person and feel safe with him or her. The therapist I respect most has printed on her business cards, "Counsel, Insight, Perspective." If that isn't what you're getting for your $60 an hour, see someone else.

As you grow spiritually and live addiction-free, you are apt to find your overall stress level has decreased. Part of this will reflect a change in your attitude: There simply aren't as many things that drive you crazy anymore. And there will be fewer stress factors in your life simply because things will be in better order. (For example, you'll keep change in the car so you won't have to worry about having coins for parking meters.) If you need additional stress-management techniques, try meditation, affirmations, and prayer; vigorous physical activity; massage and other bodywork; relaxation procedures such as yoga (the breathing practices, in particular) or self-hypnosis; play and laughter; sitting with your feelings (see page 37); talking out feelings with another person; spending time in nature or with a companion animal; or keeping a journal.

These are wonderful practices, but I don't like the term *stress management*. We tend to manage everything far too much. I see gentle helpers like meditation and relaxation less as stress managers than as stress embracers. The best information I was given for dealing with my daughter's fussiness during her "terrible two's" was to take her into my arms when she was out of control and hold her securely. It was sometimes a tricky maneuver—if you've known tearful two-year-olds, you know that they can be pretty slippery—but it nearly always worked. Her sobs would melt into whimpers, her muscles would relax, and we'd be able to rock and talk, pet the kitty, and put the crisis behind us.

The techniques listed here can embrace stress in much the same way that one can embrace a troubled child. When I do this for myself, whatever is causing me stress seems to loosen up and let go. When I take the time to use any of the calming techniques available to me, I see that I'm really embracing that child-like part of me. When that part in any of us is comforted and content, we really don't need much more.

THE LOVE AND POWER OF COMPASSION

COMPASSION IS ONE GIFT OF A LOVE-POWERED LIFE. If we were truly separate from one another, separate from the Earth, and separate from our spiritual essence, selfishness would be the winning ticket. Compassion—that ability to "feel with" others—would be expendable. It could even be a detriment. As things really are, each of us only appears to be an independent entity. At a very basic level, we are a part of all human beings and a part of everything that exists. It benefits us to think of others, not because there is some cosmic tally system of rewards and punishments but because the compassion we share with each other is shared with the whole, ourselves included. For recovering food addicts, compassion is indispensable because it is the opposite of selfishness. Addiction cannot exist without selfishness, just as fire cannot exist without oxygen.

Selfishness manifests itself in many ways. Surprisingly enough, self-effacement, self-denial, and self-hate are among them. These are not only negative and damaging, they're self-centered. Compassion, on the other hand, extends to those around us as well as to ourselves. It is all-inclusive. Our underlying connectedness makes this so.

In spite of the apparent separateness of everyone and everything, numerous individuals and even entire civilizations have seen a fundamental unity within this diversity. The Native American world view has traditionally been one that has celebrated the interconnectedness of all life. Aldous Huxley, the author of dozens of short story collections and essays, called this the Perennial

Philosophy and wrote a book by that name.

Many people have come to an inner sense of this oneness, having had what we refer to as a spiritual experience, a unique state in which a person is intensely aware of the unity—and some would say the divinity—of all life. We call these people mystics and think of them as different from the rest of us. I see them only as people who have traveled to a place I've never been and came back different.

Not only have visionaries and idealists glimpsed this oneness of all life but many contemporary scientists have as well. From the viewpoint of the new physics, Fritjof Capra, Ph.D., author of *The Tao of Physics,* writes, "Quantum theory forces us to see the universe not as a collection of physical objects but rather as a complicated web of relations between the various parts of a unified whole."

Compassion may be expressed in a variety of ways. When it becomes a factor in your food choices, as it is in a Love-powered diet, get ready for amazing things to happen.

Choosing foods based on our relationship with the Earth and our relationship with others makes compassionate living more than just a food issue. It touches every facet of our lives. Compassion is an attitude with actions and resultant consequences. You may take compassionate action in ways that I haven't discovered yet. I may have come upon some areas of compassionate living that are new to you.

We all benefit when we can learn from each other. Among the ways you can incorporate more compassion into your life are the following:

Revise your definition of compassion. It isn't pity. It is not the province of a Goody Two-shoes or a bleeding heart. The compassionate person has simply developed an aptitude for caring, like the artist develops an aptitude for painting. The only difference is that as human beings we all have an innate talent for compassion.

Enlarge your capacity to nurture. We nurture ourselves and others when we accept that all people and all creatures have needs, that it is all right to have needs, and that doing what we can to meet them can be fulfilling.

Retire as a judge. Stepping down from the bench relieves us of the responsibility of evaluating every person and situation in our lives.

Release your expectations. Addictive people often think that they can save the world. We can't. We can do our part and release the rest.

Permit other people to be themselves. Just because you change doesn't mean everyone else wants to. Resist the temptation to help them out too much. Perhaps their opportunity to grow hasn't happened yet.

Listen. Without giving advice, parading your wisdom, or trying to fix anything, listen to the other person. Also listen to your body and to nature.

Extend your circle of compassion. "Until he extends the circle of his compassion to all living things, man will not himself find peace," wrote Albert Schweitzer, author of *The Spiritual Life.*

Realize that little things count. One phone call can make a person's day. Recycling one aluminum can saves enough energy to run a television for three hours. Little things add up.

Become a compassionate consumer. We make purchases because a certain product is our regular brand, it catches our eye, or it's on sale this week. Compassion can be as much an influence as habit, eye appeal, and price. Our buying habits have far-reaching effects. When we shop compassionately, we're also shopping consciously, freeing ourselves from the hypnotic lure of the marketplace.

Treat yourself with compassion. When we ease up on ourselves, we tend to ease up on those around us. We expect less perfection from people and circumstances and appreciate the beauty in imperfect people and things.

Reflect from time to time on how your actions affect the whole. This not only shows you areas in which you might do better but also serves as a reminder of the many areas in which you're doing very well. Seeing the beneficial impact that your life is having can make you feel exceptionally good about who you are.

Make compassionate living an adventure. Be a part of the upward progression of the universe (as a teacher of mine liked to call it) and make life interesting, meaningful, and lots of fun.

Trust that you'll be okay. The ability to show compassion is impeded by inordinate worrying about our own welfare. The antidote is faith. If faith sounds too much like Sunday morning, try the definition from author and physician C. Norman Shealy, M.D., Ph.D., of the Shealy Institute for Comprehensive Health Care: "Believing that the purpose of life is good even if you can't figure it out."

Take the time to reach out. Everyone is busy, but our success doesn't necessarily correspond with how busy we are. Some of the most successful people are the least hurried. They know that there is time for what's important, and sharing compassion is important.

Give your compassion the opportunity to grow. Don't push yourself into actions that seem absurd to you. If, however, you find yourself catching an uninvited insect and releasing it outside instead of reaching for the bug spray, don't think that you've lost your mind. You may instead have found your heart.

As we begin to see some of these actions being taken automatically and as we encourage ourselves to take other actions, it is crucial to remember that compassion is not a form of barter. It's not a way to get Brownie points with God. The fact that we're capable of living compassionately is itself a gift. When my primary avocation was binge eating, I was in awe of the people who seemed so effortlessly able to be available for others. They were literacy volunteers. They provided foster homes for stray dogs and cats. They planted flowers.

It was the ones who planted flowers that fascinated me most. They always seemed to be saying something like, "My begonias are out!" I never knew if they were onto something—I mean, is it really wonderful to have your begonias out?—or if they merely got a kick out of petty foolishness. It was when they brought cuttings around so everybody else could grow begonias that I got an inkling of what was going on. Planting something in the earth is a true show of compassion. Watering and waiting while a flower blooms in its own time and then appreciating and sharing its beauty with others is about as sublime a chain of events as this world can offer.

I wanted this in my life, but when I tried to emulate these people, it never worked. It was like trying to stay on a diet. My version of compassionate living was to compulsively care for the rest of the world, ignore my own needs, and end up feeling resentful. Or I would throw myself into causes and burn out before the first victory because I had written so many letters, made so many phone calls, and attended so many committee meetings that I was too tired to care what happened. It became apparent that freedom from addiction, healthy balance, and the compassion that would make my life count for something would not result from my best efforts at self-improvement. Freedom, balance, and compassion were already within me, as they are in you. In loving yourself thin, they blossom, along with the begonias.

THE EXERCISE OBSESSION

OBSESSIVE EXERCISE IS ANY FITNESS program that interferes with your life as a whole. New exercisers are often overzealous, but they soon become more moderate. Obsessive exercise, however, is not self-correcting. Like other addictions, it is progressive.

Knowing whether you're exercising obsessively or just enthusiastically can be a tough call. A person who works out six times a week but can skip a day without regret is probably not obsessed with exercise. But another person exercising six days a week may rigidly stick to that workout schedule even when it means exacerbating an injury, rescheduling important business appointments, or missing a son's or daughter's first softball game of the season. That's interfering with life.

If you're accustomed to exercising regularly, you feel a letdown without it. Your body and mind get used to steady doses of endorphins, the "feel-good" chemicals that your system produces in response to vigorous activity. Your muscles become accustomed to exercising daily or three times a week, or whatever your schedule is. And if you're doing exercise that you really like, you look forward to it as a form of recreation as well. All these motivators are good because they make it easier to incorporate exercise into your life.

Obsessive exercise, however, is not motivated by wanting to feel good, having eager muscles, or enjoying recreation. It comes from believing that your worth is dependent upon how much you exercise. Many of us, particularly if we have been overweight or thought that we have been, measure our worth with a scale, skin-fold calipers, and a tape around the waist. The size, shape, and firmness of our bodies seem to be the most important indicators of our value as human beings. If we believe this, we no longer choose to exercise. We're forced to exercise. The exercise is healthy, but the motivation isn't. When we're pushed to exert ourselves beyond a reasonable point, the physical activity itself can become detrimental.

Here are some questions to ask yourself if you think that you may be an obsessive exerciser.

- Do I exercise when I'm injured or sick?
- Do I exercise when it means skimping on sleep?
- Do I cancel social or professional plans in order to exercise?
- Do I skip meals to exercise (with or without compulsively eating later to compensate)?
- Do I feel guilty when I miss a workout?
- Do I keep close track of the results that exercise is having on my body by weighing and measuring myself persistently?
- Do I yo-yo from exercising a lot (7 to 15 or more hours a week) to not at all?
- Do I exercise to make up for overeating?

If you answered affirmatively to two or more of these questions, you may be an exercise-obsessive.

If you answered the last question affirmatively, you could be exercising to rationalize binge eating. This is particularly dangerous because using exercise as an excuse to binge makes physical activity part of your food (and/or dieting) addiction. Juggling overeating (and/or undereating) with compulsive exercise is a trying performance. The inner changes that will arrest food addiction will do the same with exercise addiction.

You should also:

Dedicate yourself to wellness, not thinness. When overall wellness is your goal, a balanced life is more important than rapid weight loss or flattening your abdomen in 14 days.

Guard against thinking of exercise in terms of calories utilized. If you find yourself rationalizing extra food or a food you know to be harmful by telling yourself, "I'll take an extra aerobics class this week," you are on shaky ground. Use your spiritual principles and your support group to set your thinking straight.

Set a reasonable schedule for exercise and stay with that. Three days a week should be the minimum, six the maximum. (Your body needs one day a week to rest.)

Respect your body's current needs. The body requires regular exercise, but circumstances can make other needs a priority. If you're in the acute stage of an illness, even if it's just a cold, you need rest, not exercise. If you're injured, you need to lay off for a couple of days or change the kind of exercise you do (switch from running to swimming, for example) until you've healed.

Make exercise a part of your life as a whole. Make some of your activity part of your family life (a Saturday morning bike ride, walking with your spouse, running with the dog) or your social activities (joining a folk dance club or a hiking group). Some exercise can also be incidental like walking to the grocery store or cycling to the office. When your exercise has more meaning than what it's doing for your hips, obsession is less apt to take over.

Consider your commitment to exercise as a long-term one. When you really believe that you'll stay active for life, it's not threatening to go easy or take a day off when you need to.

Use some of your exercise time for nonexerting activities such as yoga, tai chi, or meditative walking. Beyond the three weekly sessions of aerobic conditioning your heart deserves, you can choose from a variety of other aerobic and nonaerobic activities. If you're obsessive about exercise, you may rail against the milder pursuits that don't seem to burn enough calories to be worth your time. They will, however, slow you down so you can actually experience your body—an experience impaired by both compulsive eating and compulsive exercise.

Please note that purging (vomiting), laxative abuse, and compulsive exercise are bulimic behaviors, manipulative methods enabling a person to eat for a fix without the natural consequence of gaining weight. If you purge or abuse laxatives, you are a prime candidate for exercise obsession, too. Your recovery may require growing beyond these cover-up activities before your eating moderates on a consistent basis. Trust the process to deal with first things first, and get whatever help (be it medical, psychological, or spiritual) you need.

PLAYTIME

PLAY IS AS ESSENTIAL FOR A HEALTHY LIFE as good nutrition, sleep, and exercise. It's an excellent de-stressor, can clear our thinking, and helps us put things into better perspective. Play and creativity are also inextricably linked. When we let our inner child come out to play, original thought often comes, too. Matthew Fox, author of *Creation Spirituality: Liberating Gifts for the Peoples of the Earth*, writes that art is "the result of play." Of course, you can lead a loving life without play, but know that it won't be as productive or as enjoyable.

A common complication of addiction is that it can cause people to lose their ability, and even their desire, to play. Since food addiction can start in early childhood, some of us never fully expressed our inherently playful natures, even at that time in life when play comes most naturally. If we want to play now, we have to learn how to do it.

I was so serious about learning to play—about learning how not to be so serious—that I actually took a course in it called Play for Grown-ups. The teacher, a professional recreator, had us hanging from monkey bars and flirting with eternity from a jungle gym on the first night. Soon we worked our way up to hide-and-seek, "Simon says," and stacking ourselves into four-layer human pyramids at the park. It was terrifying, but it was great.

In that class I learned that it isn't only overeaters who can have trouble with play. A lot of people are simply addicted to adulthood. With a strictly adult mind-set, play is extraneous, useless, nonproductive, a waste of time. It can even be a little scary.

As science writer K. C. Cole once stated in a *New York Times* article, "Play is out of control. In real play, we try things just to see what happens. In other words, we take risks." In adult-only thinking, risk is justified in business deals, the stock market, and if someone is drowning, but to risk making a fool of oneself with a Frisbee—you must be kidding!

So don't start with a Frisbee. Start where you're almost comfortable. My play-class teacher did warn against card games, board games, and sports at the beginning since they're taken way too seriously.

Beyond that, it's up to you. Here are some suggestions for gently re-entering the world of play.

Develop a better opinion of goofing off. A lot us have trouble with play because we really believe that there's something wrong about not constantly working, worrying, eating, exercising, or being in some other way purposefully occupied.

Rethink the idea of payoffs. It's true that play does good things for the mind and body, but it interferes with genuine playfulness if you're thinking, "This game of tag with my kid is reducing my work-related anxieties, developing a closer parent/child bond, and firming my quadriceps muscles."

Come at play through the back door. Befriend its cousin, laughter. Get some humor into your life every day. Read the comics. See a really funny movie. When you laugh, you're enjoying yourself without inhibitions. The same thing happens in play.

Observe the play experts: children and animals. After a while, you may even want to join in their games.

Cultivate friends who are playful by nature. They're the ones who seem to take life lightly. When you look for them, you'll find them.

Liberate your own playfulness. If you feel like singing when you walk, sing when you walk. They did it in Rogers and Hammerstein musicals all the time.

Take a playful attitude into the rest of your life. This isn't to say that there aren't times to be serious, but a person who knows how to play realizes that most things aren't nearly as serious as we make them. Because that person doesn't see every incident as infinitely grave, he or she can be most effective in those situations which truly are.

TEN
Forever After

N A WEIGHT-LOSS BOOK, THIS WOULD BE THE CHAPTER ON MAINTENANCE, on keeping it off. In loving yourself thin, however, these terms have little relevance. Maintenance implies continual, even laborious, upkeep, as in "The house was okay; it was the maintenance that killed us." And "keeping it off" is, if you think about it, a rather bizarre phrase. The implication is that fat reserves already burned for energy are somehow waiting to jump back on you like a friendly pup unless you're vigilant about "keeping it off."

Things can be different now. First of all, your job is not to maintain a weight loss: Only 2 percent of people who lose over 25 pounds keep from regaining the weight within seven years. Why go with odds like that? Instead, have as your job maintaining your spiritual connection. Then your Higher Power stays in charge and you stay addiction-free one day at a time. The old odds become meaningless because your weight maintenance will be on a completely different basis.

Besides, now there is no weight-loss diet to be followed by a maintenance diet. Reasonable eating is reasonable eating. If you're normally a 130-pound woman and you eat what a 130-pound woman needs, you will eventually reach 130 pounds, whether you start at 135 or 150 or 300. You don't have to eat any differently when your weight reaches a certain point. There are also no formerly verboten foods to add back when your body is at a size that pleases you. The only foods you've chosen not to eat are those that are not loving to yourself and/or someone else in your opinion. Being at a comfortable body weight isn't going to cause you to love yourself or others less.

But the most important reason that weight maintenance is not really an issue is that weight itself was never really the issue. It was an aftereffect. Loving yourself thin deals with causes. These are the facts.

Addictive eating is an illness. It can recur. When conditions invite it, it will recur, regardless of body size.

Like other addictions, this one has a spiritual solution. It involves surrender to a loving Higher Power, cleaning up our lives in general, and helping others.

Living in this solution on a daily basis will prevent circumstances from developing that are conducive to relapse.

Living in the solution means continuing what works to help you live addiction-free.

Practicing the last three of the Twelve Steps on an ongoing basis is an excellent way to ensure the spiritual growth that crowds out obsession. Those steps involve continued personal inventory, prayer and meditation, sharing with others, and incorporating spiritual principles into all aspects of living. It's wise to make these steps a part of everyday activities even after you are thin. And remember that *thin* doesn't mean having a body like a model's—at least not in this book: It means having a body you're comfortable with.

The tricky part about going on with recovery when your body is the way you want it is that society has instilled in us the belief that food problems belong to fat people. In this instance, ignore society. It has not yet permeated the collective consciousness of humanity that food addiction is a disease of the spirit that has various emotional and physical ramifications. We can focus so intently on what we're eating or how much we're eating that the disease of food addiction can color our lives whether we're overeating or not. This is the food obsession that keeps us from dealing with our feelings and with real life.

Coming to grips with feelings through our spirituality and sharing with others can also be sidetracked if we're mirror-conscious. We can't take appearances too seriously. I once read about a movie star who said that he keeps his sanity (and his humility) by not putting much stock in his own press releases. Like him, we're better off not extrapolating from our success in eating rationally and living in a healthy body assumptions that aren't valid—for instance, that this is actually *our* success. We do take positive action and we can be proud of that, but we don't engineer our transformation. That's what our Higher Power does.

To better understand how this works, here's a marble analogy that an overeater with a strong recovery once used to explain it to me: "When I was just beginning to come to grips with my food addiction, I got an invisible marble bag with no marbles in it. After a while, I realized that the floor around me was covered with marbles of all sizes and colors. I started looking at them and realized that one was the cigarette marble. I picked it up, looked at it, and thought to myself that since I no longer chose to smoke, I could put that marble in the bag. Then I saw the alcohol marble and since I don't choose to drink today, I put that in the bag. I picked up the sugar marble and also placed that one in the bag, then more foods that I feel better not eating were put away.

"I then looked around for character defects that I had been practicing all my life. By this time, I'd become aware of many of them and had let them be removed, so I put the marbles for lying and gossiping and some other things in the bag. It goes on and on. When I'm doing what I need to do and letting God do for me what I can't do for myself, the string is drawn tight on that bag of marbles and I'm enjoying life just as it is, not expecting, not anticipating, just enjoying.

"Sometimes I stop doing some of the things that ensure good recovery, like reading literature that would help me, writing down my feelings, going to meetings, sharing my secrets, talking with others, and letting God be in charge of my life. Then some of the marbles start to roll out of the bag. At first I don't even realize it, but once I become aware, I can leave the marbles out to trip over or I can choose to pick them up and go back to what works. It isn't a bad thing that the marbles start to roll out: The trouble comes when I forget where they belong."

The ability to notice when we start to lose our marbles (so to speak) is the key to a lifelong reality of freedom from the food fix. If we could keep perfectly in tune with our Higher Power at all times, we wouldn't have to do anything else. But perfection among humans is rare at best, and trying to be perfect (instead of perfectly human) is a thankless task. We can, however, do our best to keep a strong connection with a loving God and keep in our lives healthy routines and spiritual practice.

If you start to see the following danger signs, tighten up your spiritual program, get support from your group or your mentor, or read portions of this book again.

- Wanting to eat alone
- Eating larger quantities than usual at more and more meals
- Eating very quickly, taking big bites
- Biting nails and chewing hair, pencils, or lots of gum
- Craving certain foods or wanting some foods over and over
- Finding meals unsatisfying (the same meals that were fine last week)
- Rationalizing behaviors with thoughts like, "I'll skip breakfast" or, "I'll exercise more"
- Turning to new compulsions, like overspending
- Experiencing a return of old binge behaviors without the binge, such as yelling, lethargy, isolation, or not keeping clean
- Feeling suddenly that you have to lose more weight

Be aware that although these signs can be indicators of incipient relapse, they are not in themselves relapses. Seeing them is not terrible. It does not mean you have "blown" anything. In fact, seeing them can be good: These signals are like the abdominal pain that gets you to the hospital before your appendix bursts. They're the warning that something needs to change so you won't have to re-enter the mire of guilt-ridden eating.

Like the woman with the invisible bag of marbles, we can go back to what works for us. It's smart to do that as soon as we realize that something is amiss. Food addiction is no game, and we cannot afford to play games with it. Even so, we don't have to be perfectionists and we don't have to be rigid. One of the joys of loving yourself thin is that it *is* enjoyable. Being honest is liberating, prayer and meditation are relaxing and comforting, and taking care of our physical bodies makes us feel good inside and out. When the illness is rampant, none of this is motivation enough, but once recovery has begun, a sort of magnetic attraction toward wellness is established. You'll want to stay with what works.

When you look at recovery as something that's for life, flexibility has to be there. Let's say that morning meditation is an important part of loving yourself thin. It's a weekday morning, you have to take the dog to the vet or the car to the shop, and you simply haven't scheduled enough time for meditation. Have you failed? Of course not. You can pray in the bus on the way to work, and you can remember your Higher Power in all the activities of the day. This has been called practicing the presence of God. You can be reminded of the wonder of life when you see a tree or a flower or a squirrel. You can feel the warmth of love when you're with your child, your mate, or a good friend. And you can experience a miracle when you eat your lunch and it is enough.

FLEXIBLE FOOD

Y OUR FOOD PROGRAM HAS TO BE FLEXIBLE, too. This is not a license to eat for a fix; it's part of your protection from it. For medical, social, financial, or geographic reasons, you may have to make additional alterations at some point in the way you eat. For example, I've traveled in some exotic places where both the food and the way in which it's prepared is quite different from what I'm accustomed to. In China, for instance, they put out a small plate before each diner and bring out courses one at a time—you're never sure how many courses there will be. This was disconcerting for the first day or two because I had to be totally dependent upon my body to tell me when it had had enough to eat, without visual cues from a standard-size plate of food. But getting more in touch with my body's signals was something I needed to learn. When I'm open to learning what I need to, I don't have to worry about food—in China or anywhere else.

Food addiction is serious and it can be frightening, but to worry about food (or anything else) is counterproductive. For this day, God takes care of my food. When I allow God to take care of the rest of my life, I have serenity. There is security in having a basic idea about what I'll eat today, but if that changes—

if I end up eating at a restaurant instead of at home, for instance—it's all right. God can come to restaurants, too.

If a food situation is troubling, do what you need to. Pray. Call someone. Even leave. My experience has been, however, that when I gave up dieting for loving myself thin, almost all food temptation went with it. I don't want to eat animals because I care about them. I don't want to eat saturated fats and lots of refined sugar because I care about me. I want to eat and live in as loving and responsible a manner as I can because I care about the Earth and about what is being left to my daughter and other children.

Another recovering food addict explains it this way: "I believe that God is extending His love and support to me and that He wants me to spread it around to those I come in contact with, including animals. For me, this means not eating them. Also, I feel that the way I eat is healthful and therefore nurturing. I'm able to be more nurturing to myself than ever, and how I eat is part of that. I want to be kind to myself and kind to our planet and to God's other living creatures."

In this frame of mind, selecting some foods and bypassing others is no longer resisting temptation. With the help of a loving Higher Power, you get that desire-level healing that we talked about earlier. When you have that, there is very little temptation to resist.

My life is better now than I could have imagined in the days of binges and remorse. I think very little about food because so many other things are more enticing. Because I have a history of food addiction, it is essential that I pay attention to my spiritual life daily, but I also want to do that because it enriches my life in countless other ways, like translating some of the general impulsiveness of my personality into creativity, energy, and enthusiasm.

My eating is not perfect either. It's best when I pay it very little mind: I eat; it's over; that's it. There are times, however, that I eat a meal, stand up, and realize that I've had too much. There's nothing I can do about it except give the incident to God and forget it. Other times, I eat some food that I know I don't need. I just want it. As long as I can eat it, enjoy it, and accept myself, I'm okay. If I started to develop guilt feelings or if I wanted to continue eating, I would need to get help—a prayer, a phone call, or an honest talk with another person about ways I may have been deluding myself.

The same system works in other aspects of life. If something is making me uncomfortable, I need to look at it and talk about it. Food addiction does not mature in a vacuum, nor does it exist by itself. One of its functions was to protect us from feelings we couldn't handle. Once the food addiction is out of the way, the feelings surface. This is normal. It's to be expected. That's why many people in recovery seek professional counseling. It doesn't mean that their recovery isn't working. It means that it is proceeding right on schedule. Until I understood this, I thought that having to deal with old issues negated the growth that I had made. Instead, I had to grow to be able to look at those issues.

A SPIRITUAL WARRANTY
• •

SOMETHING THAT ALL RECOVERING FOOD ADDICTS (and anyone else who loses weight) have to look at is body image. How thin is thin enough? You can get some arbitrary weight from a chart or a memory ("I was 115 pounds on prom night ...") but I firmly believe that your body has the wisdom to settle at the weight necessary for its optimal functioning. If you exercise regularly, your body will be less fat than it would be at the same weight if you were sedentary. In any case, you will reach and stay at the size that is right for you by living according to the principles outlined in this book. When you change your diet not with a specific goal weight in mind but because your life and your world will be better when you do, your body will take it from there.

This may be the most difficult area of all in which to trust your Higher Power. I can remember hearing a talk by someone I greatly admired about trusting in the will of a loving God. I believed that God was loving, and I had long discarded the concept that tragedy and punishment were the ways that God's will manifested in my life. I just thought that God couldn't possibly understand about my body. I felt then that I had to be really slender and have those muscles that show, not big ones, just the kind that are apparent because they're taut and aren't competing with fat for visual attention. I also had a goal weight that was as unchangeable as my date of birth or my Social Security number.

Well, I got to my goal weight. Then I went below my goal weight. Then I went well above it. Finally I gave up the fight. In recovery my body found a weight at which it's comfortable. It is slightly more than my old goal weight and a lot less than what I weighed when I insisted that the number I had chosen on the scale was the only one that I'd accept. I have no ironclad guarantee that I will never gain weight, but my body (and anything else that concerns me) is under a sort of spiritual warranty. The manufacturer takes care of it. The warranty is only invalid if I'm turning to food instead of turning to God. Today's freedom, today's spirituality, and today's contentment are that all any of us gets. As we live in the way that makes these available to us, we have every right to trust that they will be with us forever after. The trust builds on itself.

As another recovering person said: "The more I'm able to trust God and reach out to both God and other people for comfort and healing, the less need I have to eat when I am not hungry. I see my trust relationship with God (and with other people) as ongoing, something I will work at for the rest of my life. The paradox is this: I am afraid to trust, but the more I trust and put my life in God's hands, the smoother things go. Then it becomes easier to keep on trusting."

That's the trust that allows the power of Love into our lives, the Love that overcomes addiction and other assorted miseries. I have a sneaking suspicion, however, that just as we need to trust God, there may be ways in which God is trusting us. There are statues and stories, gardens and quilts, and friendships and forgiveness that might never exist if we don't create them. There are people and animals and forests and rivers asking for our love and care. It could be that as we trust in our Higher Power to keep us free from obsession one day after another, our Higher Power is trusting in us to form the friendships and plant the gardens.

It's a collective effort, an effort that doesn't leave much time for agonizing over what to have for dinner or what you think of your thighs. Your dinner will be delicious, and your thighs will be just fine. The things you have to attend to are simply more important, more appealing, and more fulfilling. Not only will your meals be comprised of Love-powered foods, your days will be filled with Love-powered activities. With this combination, you will like living in your body, and you will love living your life.

ART APPRECIATION

SOME OF THE MODELS IN FASHION magazines have beautiful bodies. Some of the guys on a sports team have beautiful bodies. Many of the nudes in the paintings have beautiful bodies. You may feel singled out in having no waist or having flabby arms, sagging breasts, big hips, big thighs, a big stomach, wrong proportions, or numerous other flaws. In mercilessly scrutinizing these, it's easy to forget that the models in the fashion magazines are often airbrushed adolescents. And the guys on the team look no better than any 20-year-old who works out. The nudes in the paintings do have big hips, big thighs, and big stomachs, but they're beautiful anyway because that's art. You're art, too—consider this a course in art appreciation.

You've probably been told that a good exercise is to stand naked in front of a full-length mirror and experience the total impact of every lump, bump, and bulge. No. That's art-criticism class. You've taken it every semester and you've passed with flying colors. Now you're enrolled in art appreciation. The concept is different. You're not supposed to judge the art (in this case, your body). You're supposed to understand it, find out what the artist had in mind when creating it, and learn why it is one of the greatest works of art of all time.

Your body is a great work of art because of its rarity, beauty, and value. Here's why.

Rarity. This comes from the fact that your body is one of a kind, unique to you. The unlikelihood of a certain sperm fertilizing a certain egg to result in your conception is, when you think about it, astounding. You are special—physically as well as in every other way.

When viewed in a universal sense, physical life itself is rare. Think of the vastness of space, the mind-boggling infinitude of an expanding universe. There may be life elsewhere, but as far as any of us knows for certain, this is it. That makes life on Earth—your life on Earth in your physical body—an extraordinary occurrence.

Beauty. The beauty of your body is a given. Nature is the most skilled artist there is, and every natural creation is beautiful. You claim your beauty the instant you decide to accept it as your birthright. We only think of ourselves as ugly when we compare the way we look to some arbitrary standard. For most of us, that standard comes from Hollywood or Madison Avenue. It's a standard based on profitability, not true human beauty. It's a standard with no roots in reality and one that is subject to change.

Accept your beauty. It doesn't matter if you're overweight. At many times in history, plumpness has been considered attractive, and to this day in parts of the Middle East, full-blown obesity is a desirable attribute. I know, you don't live in Renaissance Italy or in the Middle East, it's healthier to be slim, and you want to wear nice clothes right off the rack. Of course. You deserve to be healthy and to wear whatever you like, but that doesn't mean you can't love yourself as you are today and appreciate yourself throughout your life-long adventure of loving yourself thin. You may not have the genetics to be thin in the sense of lean and rippled, but you can be thin in the sense of healthy and attractive.

Value. Whether you like your body or not, it is of great value to you and to the people who love and depend upon you. Appreciate it. Even talk to it. Say something like, "Body, you and I have been through a lot. I have a food addiction so you've been put through tough times along with me. But I'm surrendering that addiction now and putting it in the hands of a loving Power that can take care of me so that I can take care of you. I've said disparaging things about you in the past, but I really do love and appreciate you. We're in this together."

You may feel strange talking to your body as if it were something separate from you, but food addicts are separated from their bodies anyway. Talking can help you come together as a healthy whole. The most important thing you can do to reach that end is to deepen your spiritual life every day.

A recovering overeater and bulimic who tried this explains what happened for her: "I can really look in the mirror and like what I see. I attribute this to my daily meditations and to my Higher Power that listens and tells me that I am not the sculptor of my form. The more I tune into my Highest Self instead of the ordinary, limited consciousness, the more I realize who my truest self is. And I learn to love my body because that's what I walk in. I look at myself and at the hurt child that I was and I thank my body for taking care of me so well."

When you honor the rarity, the beauty, and the value of your body, you find that art appreciation can be a snap course.

FOREVER AFTER

1. Never forget that food addiction is a disease. It can reactivate if you cease to nurture its spiritual solution.

2. Be honest in all areas of your life, especially about your food and your thoughts about food.

3. Stay with your support group, both for what it gives you and for what you bring to it. There and elsewhere, cultivate friendships with positive, accepting people.

4. Keep up your spiritual practices, especially the last three of the Twelve Steps, which deal with continued personal inventory, prayer and meditation, sharing recovery, and practicing these principles in all your affairs.

5. Cherish your body. It is beautiful. If you can't accept your body as it is, get help from people who have accepted theirs.

6. Look out for the signs that your spiritual life may need your attention and make the necessary changes.

7. Give your continued health as a whole person a high priority. This includes your physical health, your emotional well-being, your relationships, your work, your finances, as well as your happiness, creativity, and fulfillment.

8. Keep your eating flexible and livable. Replace punitive diets with healthful, life-affirming eating habits. Avoid animal foods to the degree that you're able to and avoid high-fat foods most of the time. Eat lots of fresh fruits and vegetables and get that good, satisfied feeling from whole grains. Instead of treating yourself with inferior foods, treat yourself well with the foods you eat.

9. Exercise regularly in ways that add to the overall quality of your life.

10. Express gratitude to God, to life, and to people. Every addict in recovery is a visible miracle. It's easy to get involved with living and forget that. By all means be involved with living, but at least once a day, take the time to count your blessings and thank the people and forces that made those blessings possible.

SUGGESTED READING

BOOKS ON RECOVERY, SPIRITUALITY, AND SELF-HELP

Anonymous. *Alcoholics Anonymous.* New York: Alcoholics Anonymous World Service, 1976. This is the basic text of Alcoholics Anonymous and the foundation for all the Twelve Step programs.

Anonymous. *For Today.* Rio Rancho, NM: Overeaters Anonymous, 1982. A lovely little volume of daily meditations specifically for overeaters.

Anonymous. *The Twelve Steps and Twelve Traditions.* New York: Alcoholics Anonymous World Service, 1953. A detailed exploration by one of the co-founders of Alcoholics Anonymous.

Anonymous. *The Twelve Steps and Twelve Traditions of Overeaters Anonymous.* Rio Rancho, NM: Overeaters Anonymous, 1995. Details the spiritual program of recovery for overeaters.

Bradshaw, John. *Healing the Shame That Binds You.* Deerfield Beach, FL: Health Communications, 1988. An eye-opening look at shame as the underlying issue in addiction and other life problems; offers the Twelve Steps as a solution plus other helpful exercises and techniques.

Burns, John, and three other recovered alcoholics. *The Answer to Addiction: The Path to Recovery from Alcohol, Drug, Food, and Sexual Dependencies.* New York: Crossroad Publishing Company, 1990. A profound explanation of addiction and its answer using the Twelve Steps.

Hirschmann, Jane R., and Carol H. Munter. *Overcoming Overeating.* New York: Fawcett Columbine, 1988. An anti-diet book that teaches how to discover stomach hunger instead of mouth hunger and live a more satisfying life.

————. *When Women Stop Hating Their Bodies: Freeing Yourself from Food and Weight Problems.* New York: Fawcett Columbine, 1997. A look into how women can swear off diets by learning to accept themselves.

Jones, Susan Smith. *Choose to Live Each Day Fully.* Berkeley, CA: Celestial Arts, 1994. A daily guide to health and happiness.

Nhat Hanh, Thich. *Peace Is Every Step: The Path of Mindfulness in Everyday Life.* New York: Bantam Books, 1991. A compassionate guide for learning how to bring spirituality into practicality and for merging our spiritual lives and our everyday lives into one.

Normandi, Carol, and Lauralee Roark. *It's Not about Food.* New York: G.P. Putnam's Sons, 1998. Reclaim your ability to listen to yourself, trust yourself, and make food decisions for yourself.

Pilgrim, Peace. *Peace Pilgrim: Her Life and Work in Her Own Words.* Santa Fe, NM: Ocean Tree Books, 1983. Peace Pilgrim was able to couch great truth in friendly conversation and engaging stories. This book does precisely that.

Roth, Geneen. *Feeding the Hungry Heart.* New York: NAL-Dutton, 1989. Geneen's experience as a compulsive eater and her way out puts something on nearly every page to help you accept, appreciate, and trust yourself more.

———. *Breaking Free from Compulsive Eating.* New York: Plume, 1993. A practical guide to living without compulsive eating, with suggestions for eating without distractions and getting beyond scale-watching.

BOOKS ON NUTRITION, VEGETARIANISM, AND LIFESTYLE

Attwood, Charles, M.D. *Dr. Attwood's Low-Fat Prescription for Kids: A Pediatrician's Program of Preventive Nutrition.* New York: Viking, 1995. A family-friendly nutrition guide for making sane dietary choices for kids as well as for parents, with kid-tested recipes by Sonnet Pierce.

Barnard, Neal D., M.D. *The Power of Your Plate.* Summertown, TN: The Book Publishing Company, 1990. Interviews with prominent medical doctors and scientists on food and nutrition.

———. *Food for Life: How the New Four Food Groups Can Save Your Life.* New York: Crown Trade Paperbacks, 1993. A well-documented exploration of the health benefits of a diet based on grains, vegetables, fruits, and legumes, with recipes by Jennifer Raymond.

Chopra, Deepak, M.D. *Perfect Health: The Complete Mind/Body Guide.* New York: Harmony Books, 1991. A life-affirming guide to good health, with a section on freedom from addictions.

Dufty, William. *Sugar Blues.* New York: Warner Books, 1975. An exposé on sugar and a guide for living without it.

Gittleman, Anne Louise. *Get the Salt Out: 501 Simple Ways to Cut the Salt Out of Any Diet.* New York: Crown, 1997. Tips for savor without salt.

———. *Get the Sugar Out: 501 Simple Ways to Cut the Sugar Out of Any Diet*. New York: Crown, 1996. Tips for eliminating sugar without deprivation.

Havala, Suzanne, R.D. *Shopping for Health: A Nutritionist's Aisle-by-Aisle Guide to Smart Low-Fat Choices at the Supermarket*. New York: HarperCollins, 1996. This is like having a personal trainer at the grocery store.

McDougall, John, M.D., and Mary McDougall. *The McDougall Plan for Super Health and Lifelong Weight Loss*. Clinton, NJ: New Win Publishers, 1983. A well-documented examination of a low-fat, starch-based vegetarian diet.

———. *The McDougall Program for Maximum Weight Loss*. New York: Plume, 1995. A guide to adopting a starch-based, health-supporting diet, with recipes by Mary McDougall.

Moran, Victoria. *Get the Fat Out: 501 Simple Ways to Cut the Fat in Any Diet*. New York: Crown, 1994. Tips for low-fat, high-energy eating at home and away.

Ornish, Dean, M.D. *Dr. Dean Ornish's Program for Reversing Heart Disease*. New York: Random House, 1990. An inviting guide to diet, exercise, and emotional well-being from the physician to first show that heart disease can be reversed.

Robbins, John. *Diet for a New America*. Walpole, NH: Stillpoint Publishing, 1987. A compelling volume that explores the positive impact of a totally vegetarian diet on other animals, our own health, and the health of the planet.

COOKBOOKS

NOTE: For some compulsive eaters in the early stages of recovery, cookbooks are binge triggers. If this is the case for you, stick with simple foods, easily prepared, and save the cookbooks for later. In time, you'll find that your life can accommodate every good thing—cookbooks, too.

Banchek, Linda. *Cooking for Life*. New York: Harmony Books, 1989. Recipes in keeping in with Ayurvedic guidelines for health and balance.

Diamond, Marilyn. *The American Vegetarian Cookbook from the Fit for Life Kitchen*. New York: Warner Books, 1990. A veritable encyclopedia of perfect recipes for every occasion.

Hagler, Louise. *Tofu Cookery*. Summertown, TN: The Book Publishing Company, 1991. A classic guide to using tofu for dips, soups, dressings, sauces, entrées, breads, and desserts.

Raymond, Jennifer. *The Peaceful Palate*. Summertown, TN: The Book Publishing Company, 1996. Easy, satisfying low-fat recipes.

Stepaniak, Joanne. *The Uncheese Cookbook.* Summertown, TN: The Book Publishing Company, 1994. Dairy-free cheese substitutes and classic "uncheese" dishes.

Wagner, Lindsay, and Ariane Spade. *The High Road to Health.* New York: Simon & Schuster Trade, 1996. Elegant, low-fat, totally vegetarian recipes from actress Wagner and her co-author.

SOME HELPFUL ORGANIZATIONS

T HERE ARE NUMEROUS ORGANIZATIONS and publications that can be helpful to you as you incorporate the *Love Yourself Thin* principles. To avoid overwhelming you with information, this listing has been kept brief. Through these groups and through your reading, you will be led to other resources as well.

American Natural Hygiene Society, P. O. Box 30630, Drawer L, Tampa, FL 33630; bimonthly magazine: *Health Science*. Dedicated to the principle that "health care is self-care," the American Natural Hygiene Society (ANHS) teaches natural, healthful living, which includes a diet rich in fresh, natural foods from the plant kingdom, exercise, fresh air, proper rest, and emotional poise. In addition to publishing their attractive magazine *Health Science* for members, the ANHS offers books and tapes for sale and sponsors educational seminars around the United States and an annual international natural-living conference.

American Vegan Society, 501 Old Harding Highway, Malaga, NJ 08328; quarterly journal: *Ahimsa*. Established in 1960, the American Vegan Society is dedicated to disseminating the principles of veganism (total vegetarianism with an ethical basis) to bring about healthier people, a healthier planet, and a more humane world. In addition to publishing a quarterly journal, the organization offers books and audio-visual materials for sale by mail, provides assistance and information for vegans and those interested in veganism, and sponsors a biannual convention.

North American Vegetarian Society, P. O. Box 72, Dolgeville, NY 13329; quarterly journal: *Vegetarian Voice*. This is an educational organization providing support and information for vegetarians and those interested in vegetarianism. Along with publishing an informative journal, they offer a large number of books for sale by mail, sponsor local chapters throughout the country, and hold an annual conference called Summerfest.

Overeaters Anonymous, World Service Office, P. O. Box 44020, Rio Rancho, NM 87174-4020; monthly journal: *Lifeline*. Overeaters Anonymous (OA) uses the Twelve Steps program to help people who want to stop eating compulsively. OA is not a diet club and does not endorse any particular plan of eating. It deals instead with underlying causes. There is no charge for membership, no weighing at meetings, and no one is too fat or too thin to be welcome. In addition to offering guidance on the Twelve Steps way of life, OA provides invaluable peer support and reassurance that you are not alone and that you can recover. Information on meetings, held throughout the United States and abroad, is available from the World Service Office. OA also publishes relevant literature.

Physicians Committee for Responsible Medicine, P. O. Box 6322, Washington, DC 20015; bimonthly publication: *Guide to Healthy Eating*. Active in health and research policy, the Physicians Committee for Responsible Medicine (PCRM) provides programs, such as the Gold Plan (an institutional nutrition program); publishes the *Guide to Healthy Eating* (Virginia Messina, M.P.H., R.D.), which contains informative articles and low-fat, totally vegetarian recipes; and distributes free educational materials.

The Vegetarian Resource Group, P. O. Box 1463, Baltimore, MD 21203; bimonthly publication: *Vegetarian Journal*. This educational organization has a volunteer committee of physicians and registered dietitians who aid in the development of nutrition-related publications and act as consultants in answering members' questions. One or more of these professionals reviews all nutrition articles appearing in their bimonthly journal. The Vegetarian Resource Group (VRG) also supports local groups, provides outreach to professional organizations, and sponsors an annual conference and other gatherings.

THE TWELVE STEPS

FOLLOWING ARE THE TWELVE STEPS as they come from their source, Alcoholics Anonymous. The word "alcohol" in step 1 and the word "alcoholics" in step 12 can be changed to make the steps read appropriately for dealing with your food problem.

1. We admitted we were powerless over alcohol—that our lives had become unmanageable.

2. Came to believe that a Power greater than ourselves could restore us to sanity.

3. Made a decision to turn our will and our lives over to the care of God as we understood Him.

4. Made a searching and fearless moral inventory of ourselves.

5. Admitted to God, to ourselves, and to another human being the exact nature of our wrongs.

6. Were entirely ready to have God remove all these defects of character.

7. Humbly asked Him to remove our shortcomings.

8. Made a list of all persons we had harmed and became willing to make amends to them all.

9. Made direct amends to such people wherever possible, except when to do so would injure them or others.

10. Continued to take personal inventory and when we were wrong, promptly admitted it.

11. Sought through prayer and meditation to improve our conscious contact with God as we understood Him, praying only for knowledge of His will for us and the power to carry that out.

12. Having had a spiritual awakening as the result of these steps, we tried to carry this message to alcoholics and to practice these principles in all our affairs.

CREDITS

In addition to quotations from *Alcoholics Anonymous* (see copyright page), the author gratefully acknowledges permission to quote from:

The Answer to Addiction by John Burns. Copyright © 1975. Reprinted by permission of The Queen's Work, Inc.

The McDougall Plan for Super Health and Lifelong Weight Loss by John McDougall, M.D. Reprinted by permission of the author.

Nutrition for Vegetarians by Dr. Agatha and Dr. Calvin Thrash. Reprinted by permission of New Lifestyle Books, Seale, Alabama.

The Power of Your Plate by Dr. Neal Barnard. Reprinted by permission of The Book Publishing Company, Summertown, Tennessee.

Realities for the 90's, a pamphlet by John Robbins. Reprinted by permission of the author.

Self-Esteem by Virginia Satir. Copyright © 1989 by Avanta Network. Reprinted by permission of Avanta Network.

Sunlight by Zane Kine, M.D. Reprinted by permission of the author.

The Tao of Physics by Fritjof Capra. Copyright © 1975, 1983, 1991. Reprinted by arrangement with Shambhala Publications, Inc., Boston.

The Twelve Steps and Twelve Traditions of Overeaters Anonymous by Overeaters Anonymous, Inc. Copyright © 1993. Reprinted by permission of Overeaters Anonymous, Inc.

Vegan Nutrition: Pure and Simple by Michael Klaper, M.D. Reprinted by permission of Gentle World.

A Woman Like You by Rachel V. Reprinted by permission of the author.

PERSONAL NOTES
PRAYERS, THOUGHTS, & FEELINGS

PERSONAL NOTES
PRAYERS, THOUGHTS, & FEELINGS

_____
_____
_____
_____
_____
_____
_____
_____
_____
_____
_____
_____
_____
_____
_____
_____
_____
_____
_____
_____
_____
_____
_____

PERSONAL NOTES
PRAYERS, THOUGHTS, & FEELINGS

PERSONAL NOTES
PRAYERS, THOUGHTS, & FEELINGS

PERSONAL NOTES
PRAYERS, THOUGHTS, & FEELINGS

PERSONAL NOTES
PRAYERS, THOUGHTS, & FEELINGS

HAPPY STUFF

PERSONAL NOTES
HAPPY STUFF

PERSONAL NOTES
HAPPY STUFF

PERSONAL NOTES
HAPPY STUFF

_____

_____

_____

_____

_____

_____

_____

_____

_____

_____

_____

_____

_____

_____

_____

_____

_____

PERSONAL NOTES
HAPPY STUFF

_____

_____

_____

_____

_____

_____

_____

_____

_____

_____

_____

_____

_____

_____

_____

_____

_____

_____

_____

_____

INDEX

G